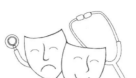

Testimonials for **Medical Improv**

I am excited to have this book as a tool and a guide. The principles of Medical Improv are explained in depth. In addition, there are extremely helpful, interactive exercises where you're given the opportunity to put theory into practice and boost your ability to communicate more effectively and professionally with finesse. As a clinical nurse educator, the interactive nature of this book is beyond invaluable.
–**Tanya Bastin-Baltz, BSN, RN, EMT-P,** Clinical Nurse Educator, Nashville, TN

As a Clinical Nurse Educator, I was planning education to bring licensed nurses and unlicensed assistive personnel together to learn about healthy work environments and address issues of communication and trust on a busy hospital unit. It was through Beth's *Interruption Awareness* video that I serendipitously found her and her extensive work with Medical Improv. After learning more about Beth's work and publications, I contacted her to share the idea I had and get her expertise and feedback, which she graciously and without hesitation, provided. Out of our exchange and the golden content of this manuscript, I was able to design and implement a two-hour session where I used medical improv exercises to bring together nurses and their assistants to get to know each other better (*I Am*), recognize differences and practice affirmative and disaffirming conversations (*Yes, and...*, *Yes, but...*), and increase awareness of the impact of interruptions in our high-stakes, high-pressure work environment (*Overload*). The experience turned out to be an overwhelming success, for both me as a teacher and the learners, as evidenced by evaluative feedback statements such as, "Most relevant core day that may actually improve morale on the floor." "Improv was fun." "Helped with communication." "I think nurses/techs will communicate better."
–**Kelly Wise, MSN, RN-BC,** Mayo Clinic, Jacksonville, Florida

Beth Boynton is a force to be reckoned with in the worlds of nursing, communication, and the use of improv techniques in the healthcare and medical milieus. Beth brings

insight, humor, creativity, and a large evidence base of proven tools that allow readers and participants to enter a new and powerful paradigm of communication and teamwork. Whether for large organizations, small teams, or individuals, Beth's work shines as a beacon that illuminates the best qualities that human beings can manifest in relation to one another.
–Keith Carlson, BSN, RN, NC-BC, Author of *Savvy Networking For Nurses: Getting Connected and Staying Connected in the 21st Century*

I always love it when people explore and re-mix different areas of concentration in new and exciting ways. In this practical and experience-based primer, Beth Boynton combines nursing experience, organizational development, and theatre to create an exciting opportunity for awakened and awakening healthcare practitioners. This is a rich body of work. I highly recommend it for ALL healthcare professionals who wish to lead with compassion or follow with assertiveness!
–Jari Holland Buck, MA, author of the award-winning book, *Hospital Stay Handbook: A Guide to Becoming a Patient Advocate for Your Loved Ones*

Communication breakdowns are often a cause of lapses in care and undermine workplace relationships as well as relationships between health professionals and their patients. This book provides simple, engaging exercises that can be easily learned and implemented to develop communication skills within healthcare teams. Drawing from key concepts in improv – most importantly the goal of helping others on the stage succeed – both the approach and substance of the exercises will challenge health professionals to think about their communication differently and lead them to more positive interactions. Many of the strategies provided in this book also can be applied to other professionals, including health care management teams, health policy leaders, and those in other industries. The instructions provided to Medical Improv trainers are clear, well-structured, and will support effect and fun workshops.
–Joanne Spetz, PhD, Professor, Philip R. Lee Institute for Health Policy Studies, Associate Director of Research, Healthforce Center, University of California, San Francisco

Beth Boynton has created an exciting and important handbook for nurses and other healthcare professionals. Her comprehensive understanding and experience with communication strategies and workplace relationship-building shows in this impressive and highly insightful book. *"Medical Improv: A New Way to Improve Communication"* belongs in the hands of every nurse, physician, and hospital administrator. Just imagine if this Medical Improv Primer were a required text for everyone in healthcare. Workplaces would be based on trust, safety and collaboration. The end result? More satisfied

employees who are motivated by passion for their work and caring for patients. Stress and competition are eased, allowing healthcare professionals to do the jobs they aspire to. This trickles down to increased quality of care and patient safety. This book is an inspiration. Bravo!
–**Martine Ehrenclou, M.A.**, author of *The Take-Charge Patient* and *Critical Conditions*

Kudos to Beth Boynton for a wonderful and practical book on Medical Improv. The core principles of improv foster a culture of acceptance and openness. When there's acceptance and openness, voices will be heard, ideas will be shared, and innovations can be found. Improv teaches us to listen and to be present for others and for ourselves and when that's practiced compassion and empathy are amplified. Beth has not only brought this practice to medicine — where improv is much needed to help improve the culture of medicine, in this book, she has given us a practical guide and sample cases making improv easy to practice. This book can fundamentally improve the way clinicians communicate with each other. If it can improve the way clinicians communicate with each other, it can improve the way care is delivered to patients. If it can improve the way care is delivered to patients, it can improve patients' outcomes… and isn't that what we all strive for?
–**Lan Nguyen, MS, MBA,** Co-Founder & CEO, ManageUP PRM

Medical Improv: A New Way to Improve Communication provides readers with a step-by-step guide to improve communication through medical improv. Through numerous examples, the author demonstrates the value of using improv as a method of improving patient outcomes through empowered communication. From the CNO or physician, to the staff nurse or social worker, she demonstrates ways for different healthcare providers to incorporate improv into their training and education. If you are interested in trying something different; something unique as a way to improve the way your team communicates, why not try Medical Improv. Beth makes is easy for anyone who is willing to give it a shot!
–**Renee Thompson, DNP, RN, CMSRN,** CEO & President, RTConnections

This book provides the roadmap towards safer patient care; critical thinking when speaking with other professionals. Putting ourselves in another's shoes, changes how we think and feel about someone different or different perceived status than us and allows for compassion and far more understanding. When participating in Medical Improv and learning new skills, such as changing how one might ask a question and instead offer an "I" statement or using open-ended statements; when dealing with medical errors; angry patients; impatient medical providers; one must stand with their own truths and be

willing to share. This can benefit the entire group and impart much understanding and compassion. The positive interactions practiced in Medical Improv insure better communication and support to one another along with understanding. This, along with cheering people on can heal and promote better teamwork and team players. This works every single time!"
–**Meg Helgert, RN, FNP,** Portland, OR

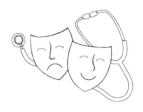

Medical Improv:
A New Way to Improve Communication
(With 15 Activities You Can Teach STAT!)

Author
Beth Boynton, RN, MS
bethboynton.com
beth@bethboynton.com

Editor
Anne Llewellyn, RN-BC, MS, BHSA, CCM, CRRN
nursesadvocates.net
allewellyn48@gmail.com

Foreword
Candace Campbell, DNP, RN, CNL, FNAP
candycampbell.com
candy@candycampbell.com

Afterword
Stephanie Frederick, RN, M.Ed.
stephaniefrederick.com
stephaniefrederick@outlook.com

Contributing Author
Jari Holland Buck, MA
jari@majesticwolf.com

Publishing Consultant
Linda O'Brien
collaboratevirtually.com
linda@collaboratevirtually.com

Graphic Design Consultant
Joanne Muckenhoupt
Psitmatters.com
Joanne@redwinghill.com

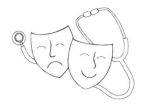

Medical Improv:
A New Way to Improve Communication
(With 15 Activities You Can Teach STAT!)

Copyright © 2017 by Beth Boynton, RN, MS.
All Rights Reserved.
CreateSpace, a DBA of On-demand Publishing, LLC, part of the Amazon group of companies.

ISBN-13: 978-1542360470
ISBN-10: 1542360471

Edited by Anne Llewellyn, RN-BC, MS, BHSA, CCM, CRRN
Foreword by Candace Campbell, DNP, RN, CNL, FNAP
Afterword by Stephanie Frederick, RN, M.Ed
"Ground Rules" by Jari Holland Buck, MA

Publishing Consultant, Linda O'Brien
Graphic Design Consultant, Joanne Muckenhoupt

Acknowledgements

I am forever grateful to my son and dear friend, Curran B. Russell. Our relationship is rich beyond measure and he continues to be a wonderful sounding board, inspiration, and teacher.

I am also most grateful to my editor and colleague, Anne Llewellyn, RN-BC, MS, BHSA, CCM, CRRN. An editor's role is a sacred one. In addition to advising about phrasing and content edits, one must be willing to challenge the author to explore deeper terrain, explain things more clearly, and engage readers on every page. Because Medical Improv is so new and this book, the first in the industry, we were in uncharted waters much of the time. *Medical Improv: A New Way to Improve Communication* reaches a much higher standard because of her input, encouragement, and questions.

In addition, I thank the contributors, Candace Campbell, DNP, RN, CNL, FNAP Stephanie Frederick, RN, M.Ed., and Jari Holland Buck, MA, along with Publishing Consultant, Linda O'Brien, and Graphic Artist, Joanne Muckenhoupt. Each of these specialists have made stellar contributions to the quality and therefore effectiveness of this 'industry-first' resource.

I am also indebted to Belinda Fu, MD, Jari Holland Buck, MA, Martine Ehrenclou, MA, and Kelly Wise, MSN, RN-BC. Your detailed and thorough feedback of the first draft was incredibly helpful. Thanks also to Tanya Bastin-Baltz, RN, BSN, Stephanie Frederick, RN, M.Ed., and Elaine Nieberding, BS, RN, HNB-BC, WWCC for your thoughtful reviews and helpful feedback.

In the Winter of 2015, I ran a crowdsource funding project called "Improvoscopy". I was hoping to raise money to film and edit improv activities and create a website that healthcare professionals could use to see brief videos of improv activities being taught and played. The project did not meet funding goals. It did, however, result in raising funds that helped make this book possible. I am grateful to the following people for their contributions and support in the idea: Peggy Berry, Carol Bridges, Candy Campbell, David Chang, Pat Cutshall, Padma Dyvine, Martine Ehrenclou, June Fabre, Stephanie Frederick, B. Lynn Goodwin, Beth Hawkes, Meg Helgert, Eileen R Hicks, Mary Kiener, Jennifer Herrera, Larry Holman, Robert Latino, Jane Leffingwell, Anne Llewellyn, Donna Maheady, Jorinda Margolis, Lori Nerbonne, Elaine Nieberding, William Owens, Kathy Quan, Judy Ringer, Curran Russell, Gary Schwartz, Peter Smith, Eileen Spillane, Diane Stark, Annette

Tersigni, Brittney Wilson, Kathryn Yarborough, Jude Treder-Wolff, and Karen Pavic Zabinski. In time, I'll continue work on the filming project and proceeds from this book will help. You are a group of compassionate progressives and by supporting this initiative you have contributed to positive improvements with patient safety, patient experience, workforce health, and the bottom line.

A special and heartfelt mention of Bonnie Kerrick, RN, BSN who edited my first book, *Confident Voices: The Nurses' Guide to Improving Communication & Creating Positive Workplaces*. Thank you for your proofing support, friendship, and ongoing encouragement of this exciting new resource!

Dedication

This book is dedicated to my dear friend and respected colleague, Colleen Poirier, RN, ONC. You are one of the most dedicated, compassionate, and smart nurses I know! You have given me many gifts. I treasure our friendship and will be forever grateful for all you have done to make this book possible. Love, Beth

Table of Contents

Foreword: Cindy Campbell DNP, RN, CNL, FNAP xv

Introduction 1
Case In Point 7

Part I: What Medical Improv is and Why We Need It 9
    Chapter One: Medical Improv as an "Escape Fire"! 11
    Chapter Two: Communication and Behavior 23
    Chapter Three: Core Principles of Medical Improv 37

Part II: Teaching Medical Improv 47
    Chapter Four: Preparing to Teach 49
    Chapter Five: Teaching Strategies & Additional Resources 61

Part III: 15 Fundamental Activities You Can Teach STAT! 71
    Chapter Six: 5 Activities for Improving Emotional Intelligence & Communication 73
    Chapter Seven: 5 Activities for Improving Teamwork 97
    Chapter Eight: 5 Activities for Improving Leadership & Followership 125

Afterword: Stephanie Frederick RN, MEd 150

Foreword

Beth Boynton has become my friend and colleague, as we both work to improve healthcare miscommunication using improvisational exercises.

We have had several detailed conversations about how to "move the ball forward" on this topic within our local, regional, and national campaigns, as we speak and hold improv workshops.

Within the last year, we both decided to write books on the subject. When she told me she wanted to write a "train the trainer" book, I protested, thinking it was too *ginormous* a task. Well, I'm pleased to say I was wrong; she's done it!

Certainly, we both recommend you take an improv class yourself to experience how improv techniques will enhance your practice immeasurably. The trouble is that access to improv classes is varied and Medical Improv is so new, classes are hard to find. This Primer is the perfect step to help you, the person tasked to improve your team's interprofessional communication challenges by crafting a beginning workshop.

Because of her training in Organizational Development and Healthcare, Beth is uniquely qualified to shed light on how to begin what you have likely thought as a daunting, possibly even *impossible* task. Fear not, the principles of improv provide easy, quick, and fun applications to your clinical practice. Oh, and the bonus? Once you learn to apply the principles of improv, communication in your personal life will also improve!

Sound too good to be true?

Ok, don't believe it...just read this book and TRY it. Beth has given a quick tutorial on the WHY of improv, followed by a soup-to-nuts menu of HOW TO.

There is no guarantee that you will get that raise or your love life will improve, but there IS an expectation that you will be surprised; you will have fun in the learning; and dare I say it? Your life will change. For the better.

All this for less than the cost of a good meal??

Hurry and delve into this book.

Be kind to one another.

Candy Campbell, DNP, RN, CNL, FNAP
candy@candycampbell.com
Award-winning speaker, actor, author of
Mine Your Mind: A System For Creative Problem-Solving.

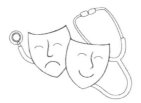

Introduction

Welcome to the emerging world of Medical Improv and thank you for becoming one of the pioneers who is using this exciting tool for experiential learning! It is an innovative and refreshing approach to promoting effective communication and related skills. This book is primarily written for healthcare educators who are seeking an effective and engaging way to build interpersonal skills with staff. It is also intended to help improvisers understand the unique needs and challenges of our high-stakes, high-stress work so they can more effectively apply their teaching skills in clinical settings.

This book will introduce the principles of Medical Improv, explain why they are so relevant to delivering care, and prepare you to teach 15 fundamental improvisational activities. Activities that are specifically designed for healthcare professionals to improve emotional intelligence (EI), communication, teamwork, and leadership, which in turn can contribute to patient safety, patient experience, recruitment and retention, and efficient use of resources.

Medical Improv holds promise because it promotes healthy dynamics where respect, ownership, collaboration, and continuous learning are infused in relationships, teams, and cultures. Even though it is too new to boast guarantees, the potential for positive, long-term, meaningful change for individuals, organizations, and the healthcare system itself, is exciting! What's more, the financial and time investments required to try it are relatively small. This paves the way for pioneers, like you, to forge ahead in new territory despite tight budgets and pressing schedules.

What is Medical Improv?

Actors learn the principles of improv so they can play hundreds of activities on stage. In Medical Improv, we take the spotlight off performing and adapt the activities for teaching extremely important skills. This broad definition comes from Dr. Belinda Fu, MD[1]

> *Medical Improv is the study and practice of improv theater philosophy and techniques as applied to the unique challenges and environment of healthcare for the benefit of improved health and well-being of providers and patients.*
> --Belinda Fu, MD

Such a definition suits an emergent field where applications and programs are evolving from a variety of professionals in a variety of ways. The theater philosophies and strategies that Dr. Fu is talking about include principles of improv and hundreds of experiential activities that can be adapted. As you gain experience with facilitating fundamental Medical Improv activities, you'll be developing a capacity to evolve with it. The experiences that you and your staff have will be valuable to all of us on the frontier. So again, welcome to the emerging field of Medical Improv!

Is it like improv comedy?

Many people who hear the word, 'improv' think of comedy. Medical Improv, although fun, is different from improv comedy because the focus is on the learning process rather than entertainment. Think about a group of children playing 'dodgeball' at recess for fun versus during gym class where the focus is on building endurance, cultivating teamwork, and developing coordination. They can have fun and develop skills in either case, yet how it is taught, coached, and facilitated will make a big difference in the learning possibilities.

As you will see, the activities in this primer are often fun while the teaching framework you'll learn to embed them in is safe for and rich with communication and related skill-building opportunities.

---

[1] Definition comes from Belinda Fu, MD in in her summary of roundtable brainstorming session with participants from the first Train-the-Trainer conference led by her and Professor Katie Watson at Northwestern University School of Medicine, June 20, 2012. See Beth Boynton, "Medical Improv," Confident Voices in Healthcare, June 8, 2013, http://www.confidentvoices.com/2013/06/08/medical-improv-keep-your-eyes-on-positive-wave-holding-huge-promise-for-healthcare-woes-thank-you-professor-watson-feinberg-school-of-medicine/.

What about improv used in business?

Some readers may be familiar with the term 'applied improvisation', often used in the business world as a way to promote efficient teamwork, creative problem-solving and effective leadership. Typically, the overarching goal is to help businesses compete more successfully and improve the bottom line. In healthcare, we must also consider more pressing goals. Medical Improv and the ideals of this book are also about improving patient safety and patient experience, as well as decreasing burnout, bullying, and occupational injuries among healthcare professionals.

How did I come to write this book?

I have an unusual combination of expertise which has brought me to this point that includes many years of nursing, improv, organizational behavior, patient safety, and teaching communication-related skills. I will describe my personal and professional career path more in Chapter One but for now, I unequivocally state: *We urgently need the benefits that improv has to offer us in healthcare!*

I am on a mission, to ensure that the value of Medical Improv is understood and the basics are accessible and affordable to a wide range of healthcare professionals and organizations. I believe the train-the-trainer approach in this primer is a realistic way for this transformative process to be introduced and integrated into professional development programs and training situations across all settings! And what's really exciting is that patients, families, and healthcare workers all stand to benefit! In fact, the healthcare system itself could become more patient-centered and care-focused.

This is a challenging mission because even though Medical Improv is a promising frontier with great potential, there are barriers to introducing it. Organizational resources are tight, the field is unfamiliar, and the approach is different from typical healthcare education, thus the expertise to teach it is rare. This book is one solution. The goal is to create a resource that you can use to teach fundamental activities right away. It will also serve to prepare readers for the opportunity to explore further learning and adapt many existing improv resources to the unique challenges facing the current healthcare industry.

This train-the-trainer approach to Medical Improv is sort of like teaching a patient newly diagnosed with diabetes how to check her glucose levels and administer insulin. There is lots more to learn, but the patient does not need to know everything about diabetes all at once. In fact, that would be overwhelming. At this point, the patient will benefit from understanding the basics as soon as possible to help them adjust to being a new diabetic. From this foundation and based on their needs and readiness, additional teaching will be more effective.

This book is a starting place for teaching Medical Improv. As a Medical Improv practitioner with a long career in healthcare, I have faith that you can bring these basic experiential learning opportunities into your organization. As you do, you will make important contributions to patient safety, patient experience, and workforce health.

How to use this book

This primer will introduce you to the process, give you tools and resources you can use right away, and inspire you to practice and build on the principles of improv as they fit into your world!

In addition to the foreword and epilogue written by my esteemed colleagues, Candace Campbell, DNP, RN, CNL, FNAP and Stephanie Frederick, M.Ed, RN there are three parts to the book. Part I focuses on explaining what Medical Improv is and why we need it, Part II prepares you to teach it, and Part III brings it all home with specific activities you can use to develop your team's emotional intelligence and communication, teamwork, and leadership capacities.

You'll also find a review of additional resources, a password-protected link to a sample handout from a recent workshop at Rutgers Medical School, a handout template so you can create your own, and many objectives you can use for continuing education. There is plenty of white space in the margin and a full page for 'Notes" at the end of each activity. Remember, this is an emerging field; you and your students might have some great ideas to develop the work!

Whether you use this book a little or a lot, as a launching pad to more study, or your only foray into improv, you will be contributing to these progressive norms:

- *Care that is consistently safe and compassionate.*
- *Patient experience and staff engagement that are at all-time highs.*
- *Teamwork that is efficient and collaborative.*

- *Workplace cultures that are supportive and full of enthusiasm, respect, and ongoing learning.*
- *Resources that are available and used efficiently.*

By bringing Medical Improv into your organization you'll be taking important steps to sustain and promote these ideals. Medical Improv could be used to permeate the culture of healthcare organizations in the following ways:

- As a CEO or CNO, you might use it as a strategy for creating or sustaining a 'Culture of Safety'.
- As a Manager, you might use it to engage your staff or cultivate communication and collaboration within teams, among shifts, and between departments throughout your organization.
- As a staff RN, PT, MSW or other professional, you might bring together a group of enthusiastic colleagues to try out some of the activities in a relaxed setting just to have fun as a team.
- As a community outreach or patient advocacy professional, you might create public workshops that help to empower patients/consumers and caregivers to build relationships.
- As one of the faculty of your nursing, medical, or other professional educational program, you might integrate ideas into classes on leadership or communication and develop curricula for interdisciplinary coursework!
- As an applied improv instructor you might collaborate with healthcare professionals and organizations to help them adapt a wide range of activities to address the unique challenges we face and critical outcomes we are seeking.

As you will see, there are endless possibilities and the effects of such positive changes are likely to ripple out to organizations and communities.

Thank you for becoming a pioneer with us in the emerging field of Medical Improv. The following Case in Point example illustrates how and what kinds of changes are possible through respectful communications. The contributing authors, publishing crew, and I are cheering you on!

Beth

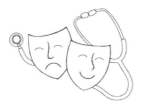

Case In Point

Medical Improv: A New Way to Improve Communication is a resource designed to help eliminate toxic behaviors and dynamics. Take a minute to read both scenarios. Note how through respective communication a difficult situation can be resolved in a positive manner.

Scenario A: *A post-op patient is horrified to see a nurse pick up soiled wound gauze from the floor without gloves and tells the surgeon, "It was disgusting". The surgeon tells the patient "This is unacceptable. I will find out who is to blame for this incompetence' and proceeds to yell at the nurse manager, 'Your nursing staff is incompetent and unprofessional and I want the person responsible off this unit". The nurse manager finds the nurse and yells at her, "How will we ever stop these complaints when you do something as stupid as that?" The nurse mumbles to the patient before giving her an IM injection, "I got in a lot of trouble yesterday for not using gloves". The patient hoped she got a different nurse for the rest of her stay. A month later the patient completes a survey with very critical feedback about the incident. News reached the CEO and she held a meeting with the CNO to investigate who was to blame. The nurse was given a warning and the incidents of running out of gloves in patient rooms persisted.*

Scenario B: *A post-op patient is horrified to see a nurse pick up soiled wound gauze from the floor without gloves and says to the surgeon, "It was disgusting". The surgeon responds, "I can understand how that would be disgusting. I'll talk with the nurse* *manager and see what's going on." He catches up with the nurse and takes her aside saying, "Hey, Sally, got a minute? Mrs. Smith said she noticed a nurse not wearing gloves while disposing of an old wound dressing. Was that you?" And Sally said, "Oh I know, I went to grab gloves in the bathroom, but it was empty, another patient's IV pump alarm was going off, and visitors were coming in. Thanks for calling me on it. I'll apologize to Mrs. Smith and let the nurse manager know about the glove issue." The surgeon follows with, "Great, let's talk with the nurse manager together and see what's going on with stocking the rooms." After both of these conversations took place, Mrs. Smith felt confident of the care she was receiving and the nurse manager found several rooms were out of gloves. She contacted central supply to discuss solutions. Neither the CEO nor CNO knew about the incident but did send out a congratulatory message to all staff for improved patient experience numbers three months later.*

Now that you can see how respectful communication can work, let's get started with this innovative approach to implementing positive change.

Part I: What Medical Improv is and Why We Need It

In Part I of this primer you will learn how emotional intelligence and communication are underlying components of our behaviors which are persistently and significantly impacting key outcomes. Understanding how important these skills are to patient safety, patient experience, workforce health, and efficient use of resources provides powerful incentive for seeking effective ways to develop them. This paves the way for learning the core principles of Medical Improv because they are inherently involved in building the skills.

PART ONE

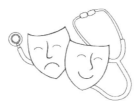

Chapter One: Medical Improv as an "Escape Fire"!

The "Escape Fire" Story

Have you ever seen the movie, *Escape Fire: The Fight to Rescue American Healthcare?*[2] The film is a compelling documentary about the overwhelming challenges we face in providing safe, compassionate, and cost-effective healthcare. Challenges involving rapidly rising costs, persistent and pervasive medical errors, frustrations and burnout among clinicians, and poor patient experiences are familiar ones. The book, although inspired by these issues, is not about them, but rather it is about an "Escape Fire".

This term, 'escape fire' comes from a story about 14 firefighters who had parachuted into a forest fire in Mann Gulch, Montana in August of 1949. They were hoping to contain the fire, but sudden high winds caused it to quickly rage out of control. In the middle of this crisis, their foreman, Wag Dodge, came up with an innovative solution as he took some matches out of his pocket and set fire to the grass directly in front of him. This fire spread creating a safe path of newly burnt area. He called for his crew to follow him, but they didn't seem to understand how his idea would save them. Dodge survived without serious injury while the rest of the crew perished. The term 'escape fire' has come to mean *an improvised, effective solution to a crisis that cannot be*

---

[2] Donald Berwick et al., *Escape Fire: The Fight to Rescue American Healthcare*, DVD, directed by Matthew Heineman and Susan Froemke, Santa Monica, Lions Gate Entertainment, 2013

solved using traditional approaches.

As Dr. Don Berwick says in the film, "We're in Mann Gulch. Healthcare is in really bad trouble. The answer is among us. Can we please stop and think and make sense of the situation and get our way out of it?"

I am excited to share a path that has great promise for those willing to consider a different approach to problem-solving.

Medical Improv, is a new approach based on the idea that healthy emotional intelligence and effective communication skills are the foundation for optimal relationships, teamwork, leadership, and culture. This is our social platform from which everything emerges. When there is a crack in this platform, such as a lack of trust and respect for self or others, we see the kinds of behaviors that are sadly familiar within today's healthcare environment. Examples of behaviors include but are not limited to; aggressive (blaming, judging, bullying), passive-aggressive (undermining, excluding or sabotaging others), and passive (repressing creativity or being silent). These behaviors are inexorably linked to an alarming persistence of medical errors, poor experiences for patients and families, and relentless stress, increases in burnout, and staggering rates of occupational injuries for the workforce.

But when this social platform is infused with trust and respect for ourselves and each other, our emotional intelligence and interactive skills will flourish. This is the exciting vision of Medical Improv! A teaching strategy that will infuse our relationships, teamwork, leadership, and cultures with emotional intelligence and communication skills that are based on trust and respect. When Medical Improv is implemented in training programs, potential outcomes include:

- Professional relationships will be rewarding, fun, and rich with learning opportunities.
- Therapeutic relationships will be empowered, compassionate, and interconnected with the privilege of providing care.
- Giving and receiving constructive feedback will be an ongoing, positive, and dynamic influence on cultures of safety, quality improvement, delivery of care, and professional career development.
- All voices on all teams will be expressed and heard.
- Leaders will nurture assertiveness, collaboration, and creativity by listening,

articulating clear visions, role-modeling positive behavior, and holding all of us accountable for respectful behavior.
- When we behave inappropriately, we'll apologize to or forgive each other and strive to do better next time.

In other words, by helping individuals develop emotional intelligence and interpersonal skills we will be helping them bring their best selves to their professional and therapeutic relationships, teams, and organizations. By doing this, we unleash the individual and collaborative capacity for prevention and creative problem-solving that will contribute to all sorts of positive shifts.

What led me to this conclusion?

There are several personal and professional experiences that help to explain how I came to believe so strongly in improv and eventually Medical Improv as a transformative teaching method.

First, in the mid-1990s I was watching my 6-year-old son Curran thrive in theater classes, camps, and shows. Somewhat introverted at school, he became vibrant, confident, and social just like he was at home. I could see that the teaching strategies and activities were helping him feel safe, to take risks in expressing himself and connecting with others. This prompted me to pay close attention to how and what he was learning in the theater realm.

Second, and around this same time, I went through a painful divorce. With the help of counseling, I began the hard work of discovering how my own behavior and patterns impacted my ability to communicate effectively and how that impacted me and my relationships. As many of us learn, nurses in particular, I was a great advocate for others, but not so good for myself. I was learning to be more assertive, trying to be a healthy role model for my son, and beginning to appreciate how helpful improv could be.

In 2001, Curran and I took a community improv class. At this point, my self-awareness was growing and I was becoming more assertive in the world. I started to make the connection between how the theater experiences that were so good for Curran could also be good for me.

I was also learning how challenging it was to practice my new skills i.e. setting limits, asking for help, learning from different perspectives, and navigating conflict in my role as a direct care RN. I started to realize that being assertive, especially when new to the practice, could be helped or hindered depending on the culture of the workplace as well as the skills and behaviors of my colleagues and supervisors. Setting limits or asking for help felt emotionally risky. *Was I not good enough? Would I be judged?*

Sadly, the nursing culture I found myself in was not supportive. If I tried to set a limit, for example, being unavailable to work overtime because I wanted and needed to be home with my son, I would get looks of disapproval from my colleagues or comments like, "I had to work overtime when my kids were little." A manager once told me in such a situation, "If you don't like the expectation you know where the door is."

I was discovering what many nurses can attest to, that it is very difficult to practice self-care with this kind of leadership or in such a culture. I also began to understand how complex assertiveness was! Not only did it involve my own growth and behavior, it also involved the culture I was working in.

I felt so frustrated back then, trying to communicate respectfully and keep myself healthy, that I decided to leave healthcare. In 2003, I started work on my Masters in organization and management. I studied emotional intelligence, group dynamics, organizational behavior, and leadership. These courses opened my eyes to more connections between individual and organizational behaviors and the natural talent I have for facilitation. With continued fascination with improv as a learning tool, I developed a model that used theater games to teach related skills in children.

Shortly after graduating in 2005, I had the chance to teach a course in *Contemporary Issues in Healthcare* for healthcare professionals at Antioch University using the Institute of Medicine's *Crossing the Quality Chasm*[3] as a text. The experience turned me 'back on' to healthcare, partly because the students were committed and passionate and also because the book spoke to serious implications about communication and patient safety. I realized that we needed improv in healthcare too and that I could put all my years of nursing to good use!

---

[3] Committee on Quality of Healthcare in America, Institute of Medicine, *Crossing the Quality Chasm: A New Health System for the 21st Century*, Washington, National Academies Press, 2001; electronic version available at https://www.nap.edu/catalog/10027/crossing-the-quality-chasm-a-new-health-system-for-the

Around this same time I began my consulting business. I continued taking improv classes and integrating activities I was learning into the workshops I was teaching on communication and other related skills. Joyfully as a teacher, I could see students take more risk in speaking up and listening as they gained trust and became more confident individually and together.

Fast forward to winter of 2011. Just after publishing my first book, *Confident Voices*[4], I received an email from my son that highlighted a call for presentations for a Public Health and Theater Arts Forum at New York University. The email linked to a submissions form. I noted in the instructions that the deadline for the proposal was for that day! I submitted a proposal titled; *Using Improv to Develop Communication & Collaboration Skills among Healthcare Professionals* and it was accepted.

In preparing for this workshop I decided to try a new activity called *Overload* which you'll learn more about later. It was supposed to be useful for developing listening and concentration skills. When participants at the NYU forum enacted it, I could see it was a profound way to validate, experience, and talk about the impact of stress. This theory had the potential to open the door to discussion and skill-building around the importance of respecting one's own and each other's limits. This led to a pilot workshop and YouTube video called: "Interruption Awareness: A Nursing Minute for Patient Safety"[5]

As a result of these experiences, the idea of combining traditional teaching methods with experiential activities from improv was now securely planted in my heart and mind!

In 2012 I began writing my second book, *Successful Nurse Communication*[6] that emphasizes a behavioral approach to teaching communication. The experience was an exciting and demanding honor and required me to pass rigorous academic standards that the publisher F.A. Davis Publishing Co. set. As part of the process, every chapter was sent out for review to 2 or 3 nurse instructors; each provided anonymous feedback that frequently challenged my thinking, called for more research, and

---

[4] Beth Boynton, Confident Voices: The Nurses' Guide to Improving Communication & Creating Positive Workplaces, CreateSpace, 2009

[5] Beth Boynton, "Interruption Awareness: A Nursing Minute for Patient Safety." *YouTube*, uploaded January 2012, https://www.YouTube.com/watch?v=PGK9_CkhRNw

[6] Beth Boynton, Successful Nurse Communication: Safe Care, Healthy Workplaces, & Rewarding Careers. Philadelphia, F.A. Davis Publishing Company, 2016

multiple revisions! It took over 3 years to complete the process. The book was published in September of 2015. The book itself has only a page about Medical Improv, but I included many activities adapted from improv in the Instructor's Guide.

During this same period, my consulting work allowed me more creative latitude and I was itching to further integrate improv into my teaching. In the winter of 2012, I decided to pilot two new workshops; *Improv for Nurses* and *Improv for Healthcare Professionals*. Both took place in May of 2012 in a friend's barn in Cape Neddick, ME. While I was promoting them, a colleague asked if I had heard about a Medical Improv program going on at Northwestern University Feinberg School of Medicine (NUFSoM). I had not heard about the program and was excited to find out about other pioneers!

I soon discovered that Professor Katie Watson, JD and Dr. Belinda Fu, MD were doing work in this emerging field. Watson was teaching a course using improv with medical students at NUFoM and Dr. Fu, a family physician, was also involved in improv comedy. Here is how our work came together.

Professor Watson originated the term 'Medical Improv' in her landmark Humanities course for medical students in 2002. She published a *Perspective: Serious Play: Teaching Medical Skills with Improvisational Theater Techniques*[7] in 2011 after several years of teaching it. Dr. Fu happened to read the paper and called Professor Watson. They brainstormed the idea of using Watson's curriculum to create a train-the-trainer program. Their proposal got a green light from Northwestern to run a four-day workshop. I applied for a space and shared my "Interruption Awareness" YouTube with Katie Watson who invited me to teach the *Overload* activity as a guest segment at the workshop! Together, with Watson leading, they taught the program for about 25 doctors, nurses, lawyers, actors, and social workers. It was one of the most inspiring professional experiences I've ever had and added to my enthusiasm for Medical Improv.

Watson's publication is worth another mention because it revealed important evidence about what medical students' gained in communication skills and their ability to

---

[7] Katie Watson, "Perspective: Serious Play: Teaching Medical Skills with Improvisational Theatre Techniques, *Academic Medicine*, 86:10 (2011); electronic version available at http://journals.lww.com/academicmedicine/Fulltext/2011/10000/Perspective__Serious_Play__Teaching_Medical_Skills.23.aspx

collaborate. Using data collected through 2008[8], Watson's students reported improvements in competencies such as; being able to think on their feet in front of others, risk-taking in sharing an idea even when uncertain, being more focused, gaining attentive listening skills, and an overall increase in confidence.

Meanwhile, these and other interactive skills were becoming increasingly important to leaders in healthcare circles because of alarming issues with patient safety, patient experience, and workforce health. The links between communication and related skills to these issues were becoming and continue to be a growing concern.

In order to appreciate the enormous value Medical Improv opens up to us, it will be helpful to introduce how communication and behavior are linked to three persistent and pervasive issues; patient safety, patient experience, and workforce health. (We'll explore these relationships in more depth in Chapter Two.)

Communication, Behavior, and Patient Safety

Researching statistics on medical errors and preventable deaths associated with them in the USA can be confusing[9]. Statistics vary with definitions, measurement protocols, and data surveyed! Yet even with variations in numbers, estimates place medical errors as the 3rd leading cause of death[10]. For the purposes of this book, there are two related and important points to keep in mind.

First, underlying causes involve human interactions. This point is supported by the Joint Commission's tracking of sentinel events since 2004 which reveals that **human factors, leadership,** and **communication** are the top root causes of sentinel events from 2004 through the second quarter of 2016[11]. If you study these statistics you'll notice that some of the numbers for different types of events, e.g. falls or post-op infections go up and down over time, but the root causes involving human interactions stay the

---

[8] ibid.
[9] Beth Boynton, "Bookmark for Links to Resources & Expert Testimony on # of Deaths, Medical Errors, & Patient Safety in the U.S.," *Confident Voices in Healthcare,* December 11, 2014, http://www.confidentvoices.com/2014/12/11/bookmark-for-links-to-resources-expert-testimony-on-if-number-of-deaths-medical-errors-patient-safety-in-u-s/
[10] Steve Sternberg, "Medical Errors are the Third Leading Cause of Death in the U.S.," U.S. News & World Report, May 3, 2016, http://www.usnews.com/news/articles/2016-05-03/medical-errors-are-third-leading-cause-of-death-in-the-us
[11] The Joint Commission, "Sentinel Event Statistics Data - Root Causes by Event Type (1995- Q2 2016)- 2015), https://www.jointcommission.org/se_data_event_type_by_year_/, accessed October 24, 2016

same. Year, after year, after year!

Second, even with concerted efforts most notably from leaders like Peter Pronovost, MD's pioneering work with checklists and the 'science of safety'[12], statistics demonstrate that errors are a persistent and pervasive problem. This lack of progress is highlighted by comments regarding medical error reduction and quality improvement from Dr. Ashish Jha, professor of health policy and management at the Harvard School of Public Health. In his testimony before a Senate Subcommittee on Primary Health and Aging in July of 2014, Jha states that, "[w]e have not moved the needle in any meaningful, demonstrable way over all. In certain areas, things are better; in certain areas, things are probably worse, but we are not substantially better off compared to where we were [15 years ago[13]]".

What are we missing? In my view, we are failing to get at the underlying human dynamics that are contributing to errors and there are several reasons for this:

- The skills involved are far more challenging to develop and practice than they appear.
- Our high-stress, high-stakes work and often toxic cultures are not supportive places for taking the emotional risk in practicing new behaviors.
- Teaching this skillset requires an experiential approach which is very different from more typical clinical education involving scientific learning.
- We don't have the resources (or perceive we don't) for effective training and ongoing practice.

These points offer compelling reasons to consider alternative teaching strategies that can help us with patient safety issues. But how does patient experience fit into this puzzle?

Communication, Behavior, and Patient Experience

There are three reasons why measuring and optimizing patient satisfaction has

---

[12]Peter Pronovost, "Understand the Science of Safety," video, Agency for Healthcare Research & Quality CUSP Toolkit, http://www.ahrq.gov/professionals/education/curriculum-tools/cusptoolkit/videos/04a_scisafety/ index.html, accessed October 25, 2016

[13] United States Senate, Committee on Health Education, Labor and Pensions, Subcommittee on Primary Health and Aging, July 17, 2014, Testimony of Ashish Jha, http://www.help.senate.gov/imo/media/doc/Jha.pdf, access October 25, 2016

become a major goal for healthcare leaders. First, patients and families have become more vocal about what they want, second, hospital reimbursement is dependent/impacted by it, and third, data shows that patients do better when they are engaged and satisfied with their care[14].

One of the primary ways of measuring and standardizing patient satisfaction is a survey developed in 2006 by the Centers for Medicare and Medicaid Services. This survey called, *Hospital Consumer Assessment of Healthcare Providers and Systems*, (HCAHPS)[15] gathers information on 32 aspects of patient's experience. As the following examples illustrate almost half of these feedback points refer to staff's emotional intelligence and/or communication skills:

- During this hospital stay, how often did nurses treat you with courtesy and respect?
- During this hospital stay, how often did doctors listen carefully to you?
- During this hospital stay, staff took my preferences and those of my family or caregiver into account in deciding what my healthcare needs would be when I left.
- Before giving you any new medication, how often did hospital staff describe side effects in a way you could understand?

The point here is that the language of these and ten other questions reveal the importance of respectful interactive skills of staff. This directly or indirectly reflects the quality of collaboration and culture within the organization. This gives us a compelling reason to look at our communication and related skills and how to best teach them. Now we have two good reasons to consider Medical Improv, let's consider one more.

Communication, Behavior, and Workforce Health

In 2013, the Lucien Leape Institute at the National Patient Safety Foundation (NPSF) released a roundtable report, *Through the Eyes of the Workforce: Creating Joy, Meaning, & Safer Healthcare*[16]. The roundtable consisted of more than 25 clinical and

---

[14] Paul Barr, "Patient Experience is Increasingly Important," Hospitals & Health Networks, March 31, 2016, http://www.hhnmag.com/articles/7083-patient-experience-is-increasingly-important

[15] Medicare.gov, Hospital Compare, "Surveys of Patients' Experiences(HCAHPS)," https://www.medicare.gov/hospitalcompare/About/Survey-Patients-Experience.html, accessed October 25, 2016

[16] Lucien Leape Institute, *Through the Eyes of the Workforce: Creating Joy, Meaning, and Safer*

administrative leaders from all over the United States. The book took a serious look at the physical and psychological harm healthcare workforce is experiencing along with the connection to patient safety. Some of the most important findings are provided in the following excerpts from the Executive Summary of the report:

- "The presence of physical harm experienced by the healthcare workforce is striking, much higher than in other industries. Up to a third of nurse's experience back or musculoskeletal injuries in a year and many have unprotected contact with blood-borne pathogens."
- "Psychological harm is also common. In many healthcare organizations, staff are not treated with respect--or worse yet, they are routinely treated with disrespect. Emotional abuse, bullying, and even threats of physical assault and learning by humiliation are all often accepted as 'normal' conditions of the healthcare workplace, creating a culture of fear and intimidation that saps joy and meaning from work."
- "An environment of mutual respect is critical if the workforce is to find meaning and joy in work. In modern healthcare, teamwork is essential for safe practice, and teamwork is impossible in the absence of mutual respect".

There are other studies such as this one from the Mayo Clinic covering data from 2011-2014 which indicates that over 50% of physicians in the U.S. show some sign of burnout[17] and in 2012, approximately one-third of nurses reported an emotional exhaustion score of 27 or greater, a score considered by medical standards to be "high burnout"[18].

The stress, burnout, and occupational injury picture for healthcare professionals is admittedly complex and influenced by factors such as exposure to tragedy, high-stakes work, bullying in the workplace, inadequate staffing, unusual shiftwork, and excessive workloads. Nevertheless, emotional intelligence and interpersonal skills can promote workforce health by helping to raise awareness and honoring of one's own and others'

Healthcare, Boston, National Patient Safety Foundation, 2013; electronic version available at www.npsf.org/resource/resmgr/LLI/Through-Eyes-of-the-Workforc.pdf

[17] Tate Shanafelt et al., "Changes in Burnout and Satisfaction With Work-Life Balance in Physicians and the General US Working Population Between 2011 and 2014," *Mayo Clinic Proceedings*, 90:12 (2013); electronic version available at http://www.mayoclinicproceedings.org/article/S0025-6196(15)00716-8/abstract

[18] Jeannie Cimiotti et. al. "Nurse staffing, Burnout, and Health Care-Associated Infection," *American Journal of Infection Control*, 40:6 (2012); corrected electronic version available at https://www.ncbi.nlm.nih.gov/pmc/articles/PMC3509207/

limitations, increase the ability to ask for, offer, and refuse help, and promote a culture of safety where trust is strong and giving and receiving constructive feedback is ongoing and respectful.

In addition to these serious outcomes, the cost of providing healthcare continues to be expensive and complex. One well-documented report reveals an annual waste of over 750 billion dollars[19] including:

- Unnecessary services-$210 billion
- Excess administrative costs-$190 billion
- Inefficiently delivered services-$130 billion
- Prices that are too high-$105 billion
- Fraud-$75 billion
- Missed prevention opportunities-$55 billion

While analyzing this issue is beyond the scope of this book, it does seem reasonable to suggest that optimizing the use of resources requires effective communication, teamwork, and leadership. Consider how the nurses, receptionists, schedulers, physicians, and business managers must work together in a doctor's office to ensure that a patient's follow-up visit occurs at an appropriate time. Different members of the team have different responsibilities that rely on information from each other and outside professionals. Clinical status may be changing, results from lab work or other testing may be pending, and/or necessary medical records from different places may or may not be available. Can you imagine how ineffective communication could account for missed appointments, appointments without records or tests completed, or appointments that could have been prevented?

If we acknowledge that deficits with these skills are persistent and pervasive underlying causes of critical issues and are willing to explore Medical Improv as an effective way to improve them, then we do indeed have *an improvised, effective solution to a crisis that cannot be solved using traditional approaches*!

---

[19] Institute of *Medicine, Best Care at Lower Cost: The Path to Continuously Learning Health Care in America*, Washington, National Academies, Health and Science, 2012; electronic version available at http://www.nationalacademies.org/hmd/Reports/2012/Best-Care-at-Lower-Cost-The-Path-to-Continuously-Learning-Health-Care-in-America.aspx

Medical Improv as an 'Escape Fire"!

Enter the emerging field of Medical Improv! Where theater techniques and philosophies can be used to develop emotional intelligence, communication, teamwork, and leadership capacities and promise a host of additional benefits such as; managing conflict, reducing stress, and improving creativity, flexibility, and spontaneity. All of which can permeate our cultures and the care we provide with improved outcomes and a hopeful new energy. If you are ready to consider this new path for change we can walk down the mountain and out of the fire together!

Let's move on to Chapter Two where we'll explore communication and behavior in the context of common scenarios that impact our key outcomes!

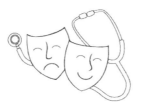

Chapter Two: Communication and Behavior

Communication skills, from an intellectual perspective, are fairly simple. However, when explored in terms of behavior they become vastly more complicated. On the surface, communication in healthcare is about reporting clinical concerns and assessing patient needs etc., but there is a lot more going on between us. In order to excel at communicating effectively and teach the skills that are necessary to do so, we must be willing to engage in deeper learning about our behavior.

Even seasoned doctors and nurses, including myself, strive to better understand who we are, what we want and need and how to express ourselves. As we grow we are learning from each other and forming relationships that in turn influence our development. These experiences are taking place within our families, our social interactions, educational experiences, spiritual circles, and our workplaces. Even in the midst of professional development, we continue our personal evolution. And as we adapt and grow, we are also impacting our workplace cultures and our workplace cultures are impacting us.

Gaining a breadth and depth of the skills and behaviors that underlie communication and benefits of optimizing them will help you appreciate the complexity of the communication problems we face and the extraordinary potential of improvisational work. This is important so that you can teach activities in a way that guides skill-building and frames the relevance to important outcomes.

As you will learn as we continue through this book, at the heart of improvisational activities is the idea that whatever participants are creating, they are creating together with a shared responsibility of helping each other to be successful. Whether an activity is in pairs, triads, or small groups there is space for each individual and everyone together, (you, me, and us).

In this section, we are going to talk about communication and behavior in three different ways: the first focuses on a discussion of limitations we face, the second looks at how both involve components of emotional intelligence (EI), and the third how improving our interactions will help us in our work as healthcare professionals.

Limitations We Face

When we think about communication as an intellectual process involving speaking up and listening we tend to oversimplify extremely complex behaviors that involve human expression, perceptions, and relationships. We are social animals; complicated, beautiful, imperfect, and ever-changing. We are all learning from our life experiences and each other as we grow and mature along our life paths. Our personalities are different and we come from diverse cultures with varied values and beliefs. It seems safe to say that many, most, or maybe even all of us have some 'baggage' from our life, family, and work experiences that impact our sense of trust in ourselves and others and consequently our approaches to social engagement.

Our interactions are influenced by these and other differences such as gender, education, social and professional status, age, mood, life stressors, and even the weather. Such differences can present endless opportunities to develop our best selves, learn from, teach, and help each other grow. But unless we are open, present, and feel safe to learn from each other some parts of what we want to communicate may be misunderstood, unspoken, or not heard. Dismissing or minimizing the importance of psychological safety as too 'touchy feely' is a grave mistake when considering how much of our communication involves critical information.

There is some fascinating work in the area of neuroscience that suggests that some of these limitations are involuntary and unconscious neurological responses to perceived threats. Neuroscientist, Dr. Stephen Porges, creator of the 'polyvagal theory'[20] explains

---

[20] Porges, Stephen W. (2011). *The Polyvagal Theory: Neurophysiological Foundations of Emotions, Attachment, Communication, and Self-regulation* (Norton Series on Interpersonal Neurobiology). W.W. Norton & Company, New York, NY.

how our social behavior can be affected by our autonomic nervous system. Way more complex than we can go into here, but his research on vagal nerve physiology reveals that we cannot be fully open or present when we feel any sense of threat to our personal safety. These autonomic responses are behaviorally linked to social communication (e.g., facial expression, vocalization, listening), mobilization (e.g., fight–flight behaviors), and immobilization (e.g., feigning death or 'freezing', vasovagal syncope, and behavioral shutdown). What this translates into is that sometimes we are giving off and receiving information that affects our relationships and the messages we exchange that we're not fully conscious of! And so is everyone else!

So let's think about this for a minute. In healthcare, we have combinations of endless diversity, relentless high-stakes, high-stress work, rapid changes in technology, new drugs and treatment options, toxic hierarchies with pervasive cultures of blame and bullying, persistent issues with errors, burnout, and workforce injuries. We also have a nervous system with involuntary and unconscious physiological responses to perceived threats that can interfere with our ability to get along and bring our best selves to our teams and organizations. It is no wonder communication and collaboration are much more complex to develop and practice than meets the eye.

Let's stay in this deeper, more complex realm of communication a little longer and explore some highlights of emotional intelligence and its role in our interactive skills.

Communication, Behavior, and Emotional Intelligence

Self-awareness means that we are able to reflect on and assess our feelings, identify what we are feeling, and have insight into why. We are able to separate current causes of emotions from past or triggered responses and use the information to stay grounded in the present.

Self-awareness also gives us a foundation that enables us to know our limits with respect to what we can and cannot do or what we do or do not want or need. This is extremely important in being able to ask for and accept help when needed, offer help when available, or refuse to help when we're not. Requesting training or seeking out resources for more information are additional ways that self-assessment is part of assertiveness and is essential in our work.

When we are emotionally safe and secure we develop self-awareness naturally because our feelings are mirrored, accepted, and explored with trusted caregivers and later, teachers. If support continues into adulthood, we go forward into our careers with a sense of confidence in how we feel and what we think. As such, we are able to bring ideas to the team, accept constructive feedback, and sustain positive self-worth in stressful situations and toxic workplace cultures, all of which involve good communication skills and positive relationships. Now for many of us, myself included, this path to adulthood can be rocky at times and effective support, inconsistent. This doesn't necessarily mean that we lack confidence completely, but helps explain why we may be shaken by toxic behaviors or cultures. I share some of my own personal and professional experiences in a 12 min YouTube called, "My Voice Lost and Found"[21].

Managing emotions refers to our ability to refrain from inappropriate behaviors despite feelings that might otherwise lead to aggressive or passive aggressive behavior. Such self-control helps us to remain calm under stress, acknowledge thoughts and feelings and channel related actions in appropriate and healthy directions. Feeling angry and thinking about aggressive or passive-aggressive actions is natural and ok, but acting out in either way is not.

The surgeon that yells at a nurse or the nurse who berates a student is manifesting a lack of self-control. Such behavior can be exacerbated by a stressful environment. Professionals may also have a history of behaving in this way without any feedback about how inappropriate or disruptive it is. Offenders and everyone within earshot may think it is ok because it has become normalized.

Another example to consider here is the nurse who deliberately excludes a colleague from an after work social gathering because she feels threatened when a surgeon complimented her colleague's technique in the operating room. This nurse lacks self-respect or may have emotional injuries that trigger a sense of rejection when the surgeon showed approval of her colleague and not her. Rather than acknowledge her feelings of insecurity and looking for ways to explore and seek help with them she behaves in a passive-aggressive way towards her peer. Immature, subconscious, or unconscious perhaps, yet these kinds of destructive and convoluted relationship dynamics are not uncommon.

Becoming more effective at managing our emotions prepares us to handle all sorts of

---

[21] Boynton, Beth (2015) "My Voice Lost and Found." *YouTube*, retrieved from: https://www.YouTube.com/watch?v=o48WD_XYqp8

stressful situations. A slow deep breath in the middle of a busy shift when we privately acknowledge that some of what we are feeling is due to a past event or things that may be going on in our private lives can help us to calm down a bit and gauge our interactions wisely. For example, if I am feeling frustrated and know at least some of my frustration is related to an argument I had with my spouse, I can be careful not to overreact about what I perceive as an unfair patient assignment. The overreacting Beth might storm off and go angrily about my work, resentful and vowing secretly to look for another job or never volunteer to stay late again. The more emotionally mature Beth notices my body tense up when I get my work assignment and think to myself as I take my slow deep breath, "Okay, Beth. You are feeling pretty angry about this, but remember you are also upset about your argument at home this morning. Some of what you are feeling is probably about that so be careful about your reaction to the work assignment." This reflection and self-control will help me to slow down my emotional reaction and be more open and flexible in a challenging situation. Will I be more collaborative? Will I be perceived as being more collaborative? Will my teammates and boss approach me differently? Will I approach conflict from a healthier, more respectful frame of mind? Most likely the answers are 'Yes'! This subtle shift in my thinking and feeling is a positive contribution to a variety of important outcomes. From a complexity science perspective, this would be described as the 'butterfly effect" and as an element of a complex adaptive system, my behavior would or could have a big impact on the system at large![22]

Motivating oneself is about having the ability to channel one's wants and needs into action-oriented steps that lead to desired goals. In addition to the self-awareness and self-control, we need to believe that our efforts will result in success, and if not success, some kind of meaningful progress. Encouragement and support for risk-taking at an early age and later helps us to develop this capacity. Healthy risk-taking is essential for continuing education, sustaining long-term career enthusiasm, and offering ideas for quality improvement efforts. An office nurse who asks the business manager to collaborate on an in-service to teach a Medical Improv activity is being assertive and so is the physician who tells the practice manager that he needs more time to provide safe care to his patients. These professionals have the initiative and self-confidence to ask for what they need!

---

[22] Boynton, Beth (2014). Properties of Complex Adaptive Systems and Relevance to People Skills Part II- Butterfly Effect. Confident Voices in Healthcare Blog. Retrieved from: http://www.confidentvoices.com/2014/02/02/complex-adaptive-systems-relevance-to-people-skills-part-ii-butterfly-effect/

The above competencies speak to the 'self' part of EI and the next competencies focus on awareness of others and our ability to manage our relationships. Here we find valuable insight about empathy, conflict management, teamwork, and collaboration.

Recognizing emotions in others involves empathy and sympathy. Healthcare professionals who are able to read a continuum of emotional cues of patients, families, and peers will be able to develop healthy and productive inter-professional and therapeutic relationships. Verbal tone, pace, body posture, and facial expressions provide subtle information to help understand what is important to others. Information can then be used to validate, clarify, and invite more exploration all of which is part of attentive listening.

Case in Point: "I can see you look worried even though you say you're not. Can you help me understand what's going on with you?" This is the type of question that might arise from interviewing a patient and result in gaining important information and building a therapeutic relationship. It might also be a manager talking with a staff nurse or a doctor talking with a medical student. We can begin to see how identifying feelings of others, which Medical Improv is extremely well suited for, can have far-reaching effects like helping us shift away from intimidating behaviors that we are all familiar with towards compassionate relationship-building at all levels. Part of the magic of Medical Improv experiences is that they allow people to progress in any area of emotional intelligence and communication that they are ready for with help from peers and leaders. For example, the nurse mentioned a couple of pages ago who felt rejected by the surgeon will have many opportunities to become more confident and secure. Just as importantly, the surgeon will gain skills at recognizing how her behaviors impact others and perhaps in that same example will become more adept in noticing and celebrating everyone's strengths. Here is a more detailed example:

Nurse manager: *Is everything ok?*

Staff nurse: *Yes, I'm fine.*

If this is the end of the conversation and the staff nurse is indeed fine then the conversation served its purpose. But an astute leader might discover more information and be more helpful.

Nurse manager: *Is everything ok?*

Staff Nurse: *Yes, I'm fine.*

Nurse manager: *I hear you say you are fine, but you looked really stressed. Please tell me more about what is going on with you. Maybe I can help.*

Staff nurse: *I am stressed. Dr. Smith just ordered stat labs on Mrs. Jones and my new post-op is having a lot of pain, and I haven't had lunch. I also worry that you will think I'm not working fast enough.*

Nurse manager: *I'm glad you spoke up. I'll take care of the stat labs. You get a better read on your post-op patient's pain and check in with me again as soon as you can. We'll figure out what needs to happen next and make sure you get a break soon, OK?*

Staff nurse: *Great, thanks.*

In the first scenario, we have an overwhelmed nurse with no meal break continuing to practice while in the second scenario we have a collaborative solution that reinforces trust and respect. We could take this example further and explore how a nurse manager who feels she doesn't have time to help staff might have two different conversations with the Chief Nursing Officer (CNO).

CNO: *How's everything going on your unit?*

Nurse Manager: *Fine.*

CNO: *You look pretty stressed. I want to know more about what is going on with you.*

Nurse Manager: *I am pretty frustrated. My team is working hard and I feel like I should be able to help them but am too busy with budget deadlines and the new computer system keeps bumping me out. We've had a lot of turnover this year and I want to be more supportive.*

CNO: *Your floor has had some challenges lately and the new software has some glitches. We've got IT working on the glitches. I think your relationships with your staff and their stress levels are a priority for you as a leader. I'd like to get you some support for the budget or extend the deadline. What are your thoughts?*

Nurse Manager: *I agree with you about my leadership priority and my staff's stress. I'd feel better if I was more available. Can you give me an idea about what budget support would look like?*

CNO: *I can call in Bob Brown. He was a nurse manager here a few years ago and does some consulting. If you can share your office space I bet he could help with this quarter's budget. He knows the unit and the process and could hit the ground running. I could give him a call?*

Nurse Manager: *That would be super. Maybe the software will be fixed and I'll be able to juggle everything better for the next quarter.*

These kinds of conversations can lead to all sorts of problem-solving and require a willingness on everyone's part to participate. And some of you might be thinking that such conversations are unrealistic because we'll never have the resources to call in a consultant or to lend a hand with staff needs. Consequently, we don't pursue them and continue our status quo that can lead to frustration, burnout, and catastrophic errors. Fostering these conversations is the path that allows us to discover true individual and organizational limitations. Honoring these limitations is essential for safe care, healthy workplaces, and rewarding careers. Medical Improv is one of the tools that build the skills and trust necessary to hold more of these conversations.

Handling relationships refers the ability to influence others' emotions. This includes being able to note that someone is getting angry and to intervene in a way that helps de-escalate a rising temper. Interventions could include validating the person's concerns, staying calm and confident, and addressing the problem head on. Each of these techniques can help others feel safe and know you are in charge.

When I used to work on a locked unit with residents with moderate to advanced dementia it was a common occurrence for someone to tell the staff, "I want to go home". It was amazing to watch how quickly their anger would rise when they were not validated as you might imagine with the following responses:

Resident: *I want to go home.*

Nurse Assistant: *You can't go home.*

Resident: *I want to go home.*

Nurse Assistant: *This is your home.*

Resident: *I want to go home.*

Nurse Assistant: *I'll get you some ice-cream.*

Of course, I would intervene when I could or offer feedback to staff about listening, yet it was striking how visceral a patient's responses seemed and how quickly they would become angry and angrier. It would only take a second or two for a resident to go from an emotional plea to go home with a begging voice and body language to an enraged demeanor with gritting teeth, clenched fists, and demanding insistence about going home. By not acknowledging their feelings, we would be ignoring them or denying their very existence which creates a power struggle that leads to aggressive behavior. The shift in energy would be palpable on the unit and much more difficult to manage. Imagine how the situation would change when staff recognize emotional cues and practice attentive listening. Can you envision how they would help prevent an episode that would require the use of sedatives and/or result in an employee or patient injury?

A validating approach, where we use good listening skills to truly focus on what the other person wants as opposed to what we think or want would look more like this:

Resident: *I want to go home.*

Nurse Assistant: *You want to go home?*

Resident: *Yes, please, I want to go home.*

Nurse Assistant: *You don't like being here at all do you?*

Resident: *No, I hate it here.*

Nurse Assistant: *I'm sorry it is so hard. Let's walk a bit.*

In this approach, the patient is typically calmer. The outcome of not going home is the same, but in the second example the resident's feelings are honored and the nurse assistant starts to build a trusting relationship. Missing opportunities for validation is a very common problem at all levels and with all professionals. In the following examples, I offer an alternative response that focuses on validating as a first step.

Staff RN: *I think we need another full-time nurse on days.*

Nurse Manager: *There is no way that I'll get that approved.*

Or,

Staff RN: *I think we need another full-time nurse on days.*

Nurse Manager: *Sounds like you are feeling overwhelmed with your workload, tell me more.*

Medical Student: *I could use 5 more minutes to prepare for rounds this morning.*

Physician: *We'll start without you then.*

Or,

Medical Student: *I could use 5 minutes to prepare for rounds this morning.*

Physician: *You seem unusually stressed. What's up?*

Housekeeper: *You're making a big mess on the floor.*

Nurse Assistant: *I have to get my patient dressed for the sing-along.*

Or,

Housekeeper: *You're making a big mess on the floor.*

Nurse Assistant: *Oh, sorry, I'm making more work for you. Mr. Jones loves to sing and I'm behind.*

Can you see how power struggles are avoided with empathic and validating responses? So often we get caught up in being right or being heard that our ability to listen is lost. Validating others does not, contrary to popular opinion, mean that the patient gets to home, the unit gets more staff, the intern gets a pass from rounds, or the housekeeper doesn't have to sweep the floor again. It does mean that people's expressions of limitations are honored and a path is created for collaborative dialogues that can help avoid or resolve conflicts, build relationships, and/or solve problems.

Using these examples, consider how more collaborative dialogues can lead to a resident who feels ready to watch a movie with others, a nursing unit that gets an extra nurse assistant for 2hrs/shift, a medical student who takes a minute to collect her breath and a nurse assistant who helps the housekeeper with a task later in the shift.

As you can see, developing EI goes hand in hand with improving communication skills, collaborating with others and becoming an effective leader. Hopefully, the links to these skills and to critical outcomes are becoming compellingly clear!

Benefits of Improving our Interactions

I like to challenge students to identify a problem or a challenge we face in healthcare that doesn't involve our 'interactive' skills. I promise you, as you become more familiar with this material you will notice them everywhere. For better or worse, they impact everything. Mastering these skills can help solve so many problems seen today in every healthcare setting; which is why I am so passionate about helping professionals find solutions that get to the root causes of so many of the issues we face! Let's look at a few!

Costs of Healthcare

Controlling costs has been a concern for as long as I have been a nurse! As mentioned in Chapter One, wasted resources are a major problem that is impacting our economy. If healthcare workers are working efficiently as a team, which is more likely to happen if they are speaking up and listening to each other, there will be less waste. In addition, necessary resources will be identified, e.g. "I need more time", "They need more training", and "We can't take on another patient without more staff"! The combinations of these requests when shared in a safe environment demonstrate efficient teamwork and assertiveness about needs is the path to discovering and addressing the true costs of providing safe care and avoiding burnout.

Patient Safety

In addition to the sentinel event discussion in Chapter One, we can explore the subcategories of the leading root causes of all sentinel events in 2015, which relate to human factors.

The subcategories of human factors are staffing levels, staffing skill mix, staff orientation, in-service education, competency, assessment, staff supervision, resident supervision, medical staff credentialing/privileging, medical staff peer review, and other (e.g., rushing, fatigue, distraction, complacency, and bias)[23].

These subcategories are riddled with implications involving communication and behavior. Safe staffing levels will in part be determined by professionals asserting their needs and leaders listening and respecting them. Medical peer review is likely to be more open when there is trust among physicians and they are skilled in giving and receiving constructive feedback.

Here are some examples:

Nurse to nurse: *I overheard you talking with your patient about hospice and want to talk with you about your communication. Do you have a few minutes?*

Doctor to doctor: *That's three post-op infections with your total knee replacements this month. We've got to figure out what is going on.*

Healthcare Professionals must have awareness of and have the ability to set limits and have them respected in order to prevent unsafe care due to rushing, fatigue, and distraction.

Here are some examples:

---

[23] The Joint Commission (2016) Sentinel Event Data-Root Causes by Event Type 2004-2015. Retrieved from: https://www.jointcommission.org/assets/1/18/Root_Causes_by_Event_Type_2004-2015.pdf

Staff Nurse: *I'm too tired to work overtime safely.*

Nurse Manager: *Okay. I'll ask Sam to stay.*

Staff Nurse 1: *I'm overwhelmed and need help. I have stat orders for two patients who are in trouble.*

Staff Nurse 2: *I can get Radiology up here for the chest x-ray. Will that help?*

It will also help prevent these kinds of errors if colleagues are attuned to each other's feelings and stressors and take the time to offer feedback and help when possible.

Nurse to colleague: *You look overwhelmed. What can I do to help?.*

After going through this section, I bet you can see additional ways that developing deeper communication skills might prevent sentinel events caused by human factors.

Patient experience

Developing respectful listening skills may be one of the most effective strategies for improving relationships between healthcare professionals and patients and families. Assertiveness is important too. Nurses or physicians who are stressed and unable to listen effectively can show ownership by apologizing and telling the patient they will come back later. "I'm sorry. I can see you are anxious about this diagnosis. I have a couple of urgent things I need to do for other patients and promise to come back and explain things better. I don't know when exactly, but sometime this afternoon. We'll make sure we get all your questions answered. OK?"

I don't think it is realistic to expect all patients to have wonderful experiences when they are sick or facing loss. But we can and should help them navigate their healthcare journey with compassion and manage tough times in a more emphatic way.

Stress and burnout

Once again the idea of being able to identify stress and ask for help is supremely important in preventing burnout. Success will also depend on leaders who listen respectfully and advocate for resources. It is also worth mentioning that sometimes there will be nurses, physicians or others who are not well-suited for a particular work environment because of sensitivities to stress. Yet, leaders who are able to give constructive feedback and staff who are able to receive it will find guidance and support that can lead to job matches that are suitable. A nurse who is constantly stressed by working in the Emergency Room may find meditation and skill-building allow him to relax and enjoy his work more. Another nurse in a similar situation may find herself more confident and happy as a Hospice nurse.

Staff engagement

Leaders who invite input and listen will be able to engage staff on change initiatives early on. If there is a long history of a toxic culture and people have been hurt by bullying and blaming behaviors, leaders who feel safe offering an apology will go a long way towards repairing and restoring trust.

Once you become aware of how communication and behavior are influencing outcomes I bet you too will start seeing them as culprits in other areas such as; unresolved conflicts, departments that are working in silos, transparency issues, and problems with electronic medical records. The list goes on and on.

Think of any change initiative and I will tell you that constructive feedback is essential which is underpinned by assertiveness and listening, which is underpinned by EI. If you are convinced, and I hope you are, that building EI will have a rippling and far reaching effect on all of our issues, then you are ready to dive into the core principles of Medical Improv!

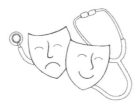

Chapter Three: Core Principles of Medical Improv

What is exciting about the principles about Medical Improv is that most of them could just as easily be rules for respectful communication and collaboration. In fact, you cannot participate in an improv activity without practicing and developing your interactive skills! Another amazing result is that while one person is developing how to be assertive another is developing improved listening skills. In the same activity and in the same moment students learn together and teach each other! When you teach or participate in an improv exercise you will get to see how profoundly transformative it can be. I find great joy in these moments and hope you will too.

There are literally hundreds of improv activities, books, and websites. If you happened upon a group of improvisers talking you might hear them exchanging all sorts of games and variations. Activities vary in complexity, number of participants, and learning goals while improv teachers vary in presentation styles. Even the number and descriptions of rules vary, but what improvisers have in common is a general understanding of the guidelines for play.

Next, I will discuss seven core principles that I believe are 'musts' for teaching and participating in Medical Improv exercises.

Core Principles

Yes and…

Yes and… is often considered the 'golden rule' of improv, applied improv, and Medical Improv and all principles can arguably fall under this. Basically what it means is that participants agree to say 'yes' and build upon what their partner offers while the 'and' refers to adding something to the mix. The 'yes' is about accepting while the 'and' is about building. Since participants do both in all interactions, they share responsibility for the story they are creating.

The following conversation illustrates this core principle as two professionals *Yes, and…* in their conversation about sports:

Surgeon: *I'm excited for football season to begin. The New England Patriots have a super strong team this year.*

Nurse manager: Yes and *the team has a wonderful new manager whom I've heard great things about.*
Surgeon: Yes and *the new manager is moving into my neighborhood so I'm hoping to get to meet him.*
Nurse manager: Yes and *I would love to have you invite him to my big BBQ Tailgate party I'm having next week.*
Surgeon: Yes and*, I'd like to bring my old football outfit and throw a few passes with him.*
Nurse manager: Yes and *I'll be sure to bring my camera for some great moments with you and him!*

Notice how each person acknowledges what the other person says and adds something more to the conversation. From a relationship perspective, they are relaxing, developing trust, and having a bit of fun together. From a communications' standpoint, the 'yes' is about validating the other person. It is integral to attentive listening and requires sharing power with others. The 'and' is about having ownership and contributing to the conversation. It is integral to assertiveness and requires taking on more power.

This sharing of power helps us transcend the old, rigid, and often toxic hierarchy into a more fluid, respectful, and collaborative one. It is important to acknowledge that this type of communication can feel emotionally risky to people on both ends of the sharing power spectrum. Generally speaking, physicians are taught to be authoritative and bear primary responsibility for clinical decision-making while nurses and others are taught to take orders. In Medical Improv, physicians learn to trust, rely on, and invite the input of others while nurses and others become more comfortable in trusting and asserting themselves. This helps everyone to become more fluid in using authoritative, assertive and collaborative leadership styles depending on the situation. You can imagine the benefits of a physician being able to make rapid decisions and shout out clear concise orders during a code while at the same time being receptive to confident interruptions from the team such as; a nurse saying, "Wait, I feel a pulse!" or the housekeeper saying, "Watch out, there's a wet spot on the floor".

Medical Improv helps to rubberize[24] the hierarchy. In other words, makes it more flexible and psychologically safe. Doctors, nurses, and other professionals who have conversations like the football example above are building trust and respect so when they are in a high-stakes high-stress clinical situation they will naturally work together more collaboratively.

The hierarchy becomes healthier because professionals acknowledge and respect each other's skills, education, and experience. The clinical ladder of expertise, authority, and responsibility allows the structure of the hierarchy to remain intact but protects it from being so rigid that it discourages, or worse ignores input from others. This respect is essential for ensuring a culture of safety where patients, families, housekeepers, nurse assistants, medical students, nurses, physicians, and others feel safe and empowered to speak up about ideas and concerns.

- Help your partner be successful

This rule encourages everyone to support each other in their ideas and actions. This concept can be foreign to people on the health care team who may have experienced learning by humiliation, studied in highly competitive educational programs, and/or work in cultures of blame. In the Medical Improv classroom, people are learning to take risks by being creative and offering ideas that are supportive of others. These efforts build trust and encourage psychological safety. In the above conversation, the surgeon

---

[24] Boynton, Beth (2015). Collaborative Leadership Can Rubberize the Hierarchy. Confident Voices in Healthcare Blog. Retrieved from: http://www.confidentvoices.com/2015/04/01/collaborative-leadership-can-rubberize-the-hierarchy/

and nurse manager are helping each other be successful by building on each other's ideas. Let's see what happens when we don't follow this principle in this scenario.

Surgeon: *I'm excited for football season to begin. The New England Patriots have a super strong team this year.*
Nurse manager: Yes, but *I've heard that the new manager doesn't have much experience.*
Surgeon: Yes, but *he's received a lot of impressive rewards and I'm hoping to get to meet him.*
Nurse manager: Yes *he's coming to my big BBQ Tailgate party I'm having next week,* **but** *you are on call that night.*
Surgeon: Yes but, *I can try to get coverage for a little while.*
Nurse manager: Yes, but *Dr. Smith and Dr. Jones who might cover for you have already agreed to come to my party.*

Notice the difference in the tone of this conversation when the surgeon and the nurse are not working to help each other be successful. Their listening is competitive and their statements are more argumentative and self-serving. In improv, we call this 'blocking' and the story that they are developing will not go very far. In real life, these two clinicians will be less likely to seek each other out for opinions or work through a conflict at work because they are sending tacit messages that they don't care about or respect the other.

Improv activities provide lots of opportunities to coach participants in shifting behavior and learn what it feels like when you are supportive or being supported. Improv allows people to build trust and respect that will help them to work together in their respective clinical environments. The more practitioners demonstrate collaborative behaviors the more they role model them and contribute to a collaborative culture. The rippling effect of these seemingly simple activities can lead to exciting, new norms.

- *You have everything you need*

Those new to improv may be worried about the need to be creative or funny or not knowing what to say. This rule is meant to help people learn to trust themselves and to allay anxiety about participating in this type of activity. In doing so people become more comfortable with their own creativity and spontaneity which leads to the generation of more ideas that can help any organizational or team initiative. With a little practice, this principle can help professionals develop the ability to tap into the skills, knowledge, and experience they have rather than being hindered by anxiety that arises from the stress of their work. Transferring these techniques into the high-stakes, high-stress world of healthcare will help ensure that all members of the team perform at their best. The entire team will communicate better and patients will have better outcomes.

- *Celebrate risk-taking*

This principle helps create an environment where it is safe to express ideas and try new ways of doing things. There can be awkward moments when a participant, myself included, who does not know what to say, says something that breaks one of the rules, or mishears something and takes a conversation in a direction that doesn't make sense. Often the person realizes her mistake and may feel embarrassed or afraid of judgment. When we celebrate risk-taking, there is a rich opportunity for everyone to support the person who has made a mistake. (I'll tell you more about how to facilitate this risk-taking in Part II). Risk-taking allows us to clap or snap our fingers and say, "I'm human" or "Yay, I screwed up!" And then resume the activity with a new approach, or start again. No big deal!

When this happens for the first time in a group it is a wonderful message for everyone to experience as it shows we are all human, we are not perfect, and it is ok, you're ok, we're ok! We can use the 'sports' example discussed earlier to demonstrate.

Surgeon: *I'm excited for football season to begin. The New England Patriots have a super strong team this year.*

Nurse manager: Yes and *I love the....wait what did you say?*

In the moment the nurse manager and others realize he forgot what the surgeon said everyone claps and shouts, "Yay she took a risk" Shortly after, the surgeon moves to help make his partner be successful in the activity and the story takes on an interesting new twist.

Surgeon: *Sorry, I was mumbling*.

Nurse manager: Yes, and *I've been worried about your speech lately. You seem to be going back in your shell.*

Surgeon: *Yes, and I have to tell you something, but I'm afraid you'll freak out.*

As these professionals become more comfortable with the activity and each other they will feel safe in trying out new ideas.

Truth and facts are not necessary

Most improvisers take this concept for granted, but I find that healthcare professionals often need permission to make things up. Conversations should still have a flow and make sense, but unlike the clinical environment, clinicians can take a break from the constant pressure of knowing the right pieces of information and use parts of their brain that generate new ideas. Since evidence exists that we use a different part of our brains for recalling information than we do for creativity, [25] it stands to reason that clinicians' brains are pretty high functioning with respect to recall but may have room for improvement in terms of creativity. Charles Lamb, a well-known neurosurgeon and musician offers a fascinating hypothesis in his TED Talk, "Your Brain on Improv"[26]:

"…to be creative, you have to have this weird dissociation in your frontal lobe. One area turns on and another area shuts off, so that you're not inhibited so that you're willing to make mistakes, so that you're not constantly shutting down all of these new generative impulses".

Even without more data on the topic, it seems like a wise decision to promote improv as a way to develop the areas in the brain that are responsible for creativity, right? We don't want to be creative about administering chemotherapy, performing a colectomy, or reporting abnormal bloodwork, but our creativity can help us when something unexpectedly goes wrong—like a piece of equipment isn't working, a family member becomes hysterical, or a patient starts to have a seizure during a central line dressing change. And certainly, we could benefit from new ideas and ways of thinking about all quality improvement and organizational change initiatives!

---

[25] Benedek M, Jauk E, Fink A, Koschutnig K, Reishofer G, Ebner F, Neubauer AC.Neuroimage. To create or to recall? Neural mechanisms underlying the generation of creative new ideas. 2013 Nov 21; 88C:125-133. Epub 2013 Nov 21.

[26] Lamb, Charles (2010). Your Brain on Improv. TEDxMidAtlantic. Retrieved from: https://www.ted.com/talks/charles_limb_your_brain_on_improv/transcript?language=en#t-527917

- *Avoid questions*

Even after years of taking improv classes, I still catch myself asking questions rather than bringing something new to the conversation. It seems I have an innate tendency to give or some would say 'dump' more responsibility on my partner for creating the story. Stopping myself from asking questions and reaching deeper for ideas has been a revealing and ongoing journey.

Consequently, questions in the clinical environment have become fascinating to me! I notice that they can arise from a place of healthy and confident curiosity or the need for information which is wonderful and necessary for continuous learning. However, sometimes questions can also be used as a way to avoid ownership or protect others' egos. Now, it wouldn't be fair to say this is always bad or wrong, but there are counterproductive consequences if/when nurses or others perpetually ask questions about things that they know the answer to or at least have a pretty good idea about.

Avoiding ownership, giving up power, and misrepresenting one's knowledge or ideas are all counterproductive to being assertive. For that reason, this principle supports important growth for many nurses. It also helps pave the way for more respectful interprofessional relationships by demonstrating confidence and revealing the truth about one's skills and knowledge. Here's an example of a nurse asking a question rather than making a statement:

Did you want to order a chest X-Ray?

Or,

I think a chest X-Ray would be a good idea!

In the second example, the physician or advanced practice registered nurse might agree and thank the nurse for the suggestion. The chest x-ray decision is shared. If the clinician does not agree, she'll have an opportunity to role model and teach collaborative leadership by thanking the nurse for his input and explaining why a chest x-ray wouldn't be a good idea in this situation. In either case, the nurses' input is respected, a learning opportunity fulfilled, their professional relationship deepens, and the patient gets a helpful test or doesn't get an unnecessary one. All this from respectful communication!

In our football example this tendency to ask questions might show up like this:

Surgeon: *I'm excited for football season to begin. The New England Patriots have a super strong team this year.*

Nurse manager: *Have you seen them play this season?*

Here the Nurse Manager isn't adding much of anything to the story. Such a situation leads to opportunities for the facilitator to coach, the class an opportunity to celebrate risk-taking, the nurse to reflect and take on more responsibility, and the surgeon to practice patience!

Surgeon: *I'm excited for football season to begin. The New England Patriots have a super strong team this year.*

Nurse manager: *Have you seen them play this season?*

Facilitator: *Try again without asking a question.*

Nurse manager: Yes and *my brother, Ralph is on the team. You guys used to play together in High School.*

Facilitator: *Awesome risk-taking!* (Leads everyone to clap hands.)

So much learning can take place in these moments!

- **Observers play an important role**

The more I teach Medical Improv classes the more I've come to realize how scary the process can seem to others who are just starting out. A student of mine shared with me her fears after class one day which I had underestimated. "I was terrified and could feel myself going into a panic mode", she shared. It didn't matter that she was doctorally educated and had a very successful practice in healthcare. The emotional risk was huge. I realized that helping her and others with similar feelings feel safe required a different approach and added this principle that values the role of observers.

While encouraging all participants to stretch out of their comfort zones I also invite those who want to observe an activity to do so with the caveat that they share their observations with the class. In addition to helping others feel safe, the class gets an alternative perspective to learn from and they stay engaged. Some people who are hesitant at first also get a chance to see the activity which can be reassuring in terms of what to expect. This decreases the risk and some observers feel more comfortable participating in the activity directly if it is repeated.

To review, here are the following core principles of medical improv.

- *Yes and...*
- *Help your partner be successful*
- *You have everything you need*
- *Celebrate risk-taking*
- *Truth and facts are not necessary*
- *Avoid questions*
- *Observers play an important role*

Having a strong sense of these core principles is essential for facilitating activities. No doubt you will add your own style and language as you develop your skills and gain experience in facilitating learning. You are now ready for Part II of this Primer that will help you become a teacher of Medical Improv!

CHAPTER THREE

Part II: Teaching Medical Improv

In the next three chapters you will learn how facilitating and coaching experiential activities is different from teaching clinical or intellectual information. You will also be prepared for teaching Medical Improv activities and workshops with planning logistics; such as, time and space needed, the importance of creating a safe environment, tips on how to do it, along with information you need to prepare handouts. I have also included a resource list for additional information. You will also find the link and password to exclusive online resources that will help you create your own handout expertly and efficiently!

Let's get started.

PART TWO

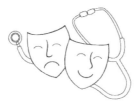

Chapter Four: Preparing to Teach

Teaching Medical Improv is fun, different, and rewarding! Fun because staff can get out of their clinical heads and stressful work environments and have some lighter time together. Even when resistant or uncomfortable at first, there seems to be an inherent joy in 'playing' together. Given the stress, loss and tragedy integral to our work, improv fills a need that we may be longing for as healthcare professionals.

Teaching Medical Improv activities is different because the emphasis is less on imparting information, such as explaining the side effects of a new drug or demonstrating the steps to using a new IV pump, and more on creating and maintaining a safe environment where all participants are engaged, can identify some of their own learning needs, and practice new behaviors. Rather than lecturing or testing, you'll be guiding individual and group behaviors that promote growth in communication and collaboration skills and emotional intelligence. You'll be calling upon your coaching and facilitation skills to gently nudge one person to share an idea, another to be patient and listen, and the whole group to be supportive of each other's risk-taking.

Teaching Medical Improv is rewarding because the new awarenesses, emotional growth, and skill-building you observe in your sessions will continue for many participants as related opportunities for practice arise in their clinical environments and with peers. Medical Improv is going to help them provide better care and feel more joy in their work! Workshop attendees often tell me days or even months after a workshop that they are still becoming better listeners or more assertive because of a particular activity we did. As a teacher, it is the kind of feedback that makes me want to jump up and down!

In this chapter, I am going to share with you my approach to teaching Medical Improv along with suggestions for applying improv into your own setting. First, some general observations I've made and then some more specific tips. We'll tie everything together more completely with examples of facilitating activities in the last three chapters.

General Observations

As a 30-year veteran nurse with a decade teaching emotional intelligence, communication, and collaboration using improv activities, I have noticed some important themes.

- Almost all "interactive" skills can be categorized as elements of assertiveness and/or listening.
- Participants will learn what they need and are ready to learn in order to progress in their own development.
- Participants in the same workshop will learn different skills.
- One person practicing assertiveness will be teaching another about listening and vice versa.
- There are many terms that can be used to describe the skills.
- Giving people a choice about what they want to focus on is an effective and engaging teaching method.
- Relationships are extremely important in our work and Medical Improv is a great way to nurture them.

The more you learn about and teach Medical Improv the more you will see just how powerful this work is. As you prepare to teach your first session, these suggestions will help you be successful. As you traverse your own learning curve, things will become easier and less time-consuming.

How much time should you plan on?

Initially you should plan on 15 minutes to introduce the principles, but once enough staff understands the core principles and you all have a little experience, you'll be able to dive right into activities with a few minutes set aside to debrief. In Part III, there are estimated time requirements for each activity that do not include teaching the principles. Also, over time as more staff are familiar with the rules, you'll be able to have sessions where staff who know how to play a game can very quickly help demonstrate to others. Add a handout, to be discussed shortly, and you won't have to say much about the rules except referring to them as needed. The learning curve is shorter as more members of the staff can help teach.

This means that with a little planning and initial investment of time, you'll eventually be able to integrate activities into clinical in-services, monthly unit meetings, and administrative planning sessions. Maybe you'll create a lunch and learn series or look for opportunities to use improv during orientation. As the process will just take a few minutes here to implement, the potential gains are major while there is not a huge drain on organizational resources.

Space and Group Size

The space you choose to hold a class needs to be big enough so that people can move around a little and in a location where it is ok to be noisy. The ideal size for this kind of work is between 6-16 participants. This will allow you to connect with everyone and offer feedback while ensuring that everyone will have a chance to participate. With tech support and co-facilitation, I do sessions with groups of 100 or more, and they can be a lot of fun. However, I don't recommend this size until you feel comfortable teaching the activities in a small group.

Letting them loose and reeling them in

I tell participants early on that there are times where I need the group to focus on me and times when they will be focused on each other. You can use a bell or tuning fork as a signal to refocus or even clap your hands. My favorite way to get a noisy and engaged group of people to quiet down quickly and bring their attention back to me is to show them the peace sign with my index and second fingers. I explain beforehand that this is a sign for them to wrap up their conversation and mirror the peace sign back to me as soon as they notice. It is really fun to see a group of engaged, lively, and even boisterous healthcare professionals playing together and then quickly quiet down at the signal! It is a great example of a human complex adaptive system following an instruction and cooperating!

Which comes first the principles or the activities?

Improv instructors vary in terms of how much teaching they do regarding the principles. When I first started teaching Medical Improv I spent significant time explaining the principals along with the many skills people can learn and the outcomes they will impact. I have come to believe with experience and feedback that instructors need this depth of understanding, but participants do not.

Participants need to know what the rules of play are, so I tend to go over them very briefly using a PowerPoint slide and a simple handout. Keeping them visible provides a structure i.e. set of norms expected for all activities. Then you can use them as reminders for facilitating play. *Try that again without asking a question* or *Remember you want to help your partner be successful* are common coaching tips you might use. Here's the list of principles from Chapter Three with sample overviews I offer.

- "Yes and…"

  This first rule means that you accept and validate what your partner brings to the table and add something of your own. It is the "Golden Rule" of improv! You cannot play an improv activity without practicing your listening and speaking up skills.

- Help your partner be successful

  It is your job to make your partner look good!

- *You have everything you need*

  This rule is meant to help you trust yourself, your partner, me and the process. There is no need to study or memorize, to be funny, or perfect!

- *Celebrate risk-taking*

  Trying something new can be scary! You may have times when you don't know what to say or feel like what you said didn't make sense. It's ok. We are all human. Anytime you are stuck or say something that doesn't seem like a good fit, we're going to celebrate your effort! I like to ask the group if they have any ideas how we can celebrate risk-taking in the moment and if nothing comes forth will suggest clapping and shouting together, "Yay, Beth took a risk" or something like that.

- **Truth and facts are not necessary**

    In Medical Improv you can make things up! Try to make sense so there is a flow, but try not to worry about being right!

- **Avoid questions**

    Try to make statements as opposed to asking questions.

- **Observers play an important role**

    It is fine to watch. Your observations will be helpful..

You can do a lot more teaching when staff are engaging in activities and even after the session is over. For example, I was having coffee with one of my improv instructors, David LaGraffe[27]. In the course of our conversation, he reminded me of a time in class a year earlier when I was doing an activity with him called *One Minute Death*. In this activity two people have one minute to act out a scene where one person dies. We both recalled being on a boat when he collapsed to the floor, dead, within the first few seconds. I started screaming and trying to do CPR. And that is basically what I did for the rest of the minute which seemed like an eternity.

In the debriefing that followed and again during our current conversation, he gently nudged me to think about other possibilities. Instead of thinking like a serious nurse/healthcare professional, I could have had a little more fun as noted in the following scenarios:

> *Free at last, the poison worked!* (I pretend to use my cell phone) *Jim, he's gone. Meet me in 20 minutes at the dock. I'll cover him with the tarp and you jump on. I'll need help with the body....*
>
> *Poor David, he should have remembered his medications, but you know I was*

---

[27] Lights Up Improv, http://www.lightsupimprov.com/, accessed October 25, 2016

tired of reminding him. All those years of cooking and cleaning for him....I'm sure I can make it to Greece and start the fine chocolate shoppe I've dreamed of...

Oh my, I've never tried driving this boat. Then taking the steering wheel and shifting sharply to the left and falling while David rolls. For all I knew this may have revived him!

In those 50 seconds, anything was possible. But I had stayed in this mode of reaction that felt familiar and comfortable rather than explore, create, or let my own ideas surface. I was responding as a clinician, which is a good thing in many situations, but there was this other part of me that was holding back. I wondered if or how my screaming and pretending to do CPR might be interfering with my creative side. *Was I afraid to try something different? What was keeping me from coming up with new ideas? Did I feel safer doing something predictable?* Reflecting on these kinds of questions and experiences has helped me to realize that while part of me was being active i.e. screaming and doing CPR, another part of me was being passive i.e. by not doing something that would change the course of the story. Improv training has helped me become aware of when I might be holding back an idea in a group, practice taking more risk, and appreciate how hard assertiveness can be. David and I laughed about the memory and our shared understanding about how complicated assertiveness can be and how memorable and deeply powerful this work can be.

Once the rules are out on the table, it is important to get participants engaged in an activity pretty quickly. One reason to get into the activities sooner rather than later is that they are fun and engaging. It is a refreshing change to be interacting in a relaxed and non-threatening environment rather than a clinical or administrative meeting. You'll see and feel the energy shift in a positive way very quickly.

Creating a safe environment

Many people express some anxiety about participating in Medical Improv activities. Fears around public speaking or performing are common fears that people associate with doing improv. This creates apprehension for those who think that Medical Improv will require them to get on stage and be funny or those who are introverted by nature.

Although you can't eliminate such fears there are several things you can and should do to minimize them. Here are some suggestions for making the environment as safe as possible.

1. *Offer reassurance.* Make sure participants know as soon as possible that Medical Improv is different from improv comedy. Let them know that there is no need to be funny or perform. Explain that most people do have fun and encourage them to stretch a bit as they would with anything new. As you gain experience teaching Medical Improv, you will have other ideas about helping people feel comfortable. I often add that we are all learning from each other, all voices are important, and that people who tend to be more introverted will be practicing speaking up at the same time as people who are more extroverted are practicing listening.

2. *Set up norms or ground rules for group behavior.* Even though there will be overlap between norms and the core principles of Medical Improv, it is important to establish things like confidentiality and mutual respect up front. Ground Rules such as those provided at the end of this chapter from author[28], patient advocate, and teacher, Jari Holland Buck, are a great tool that you can use to illustrate your expectations and ask for the group to acknowledge and commit to. They also serve as a reference point if/when any inappropriate behavior needs to be addressed.

   If you are working with a group who are generally respectful, you may simply remind them of norms verbally. If you suspect or know that you are working with a toxic culture and/or individuals who have a reputation for being disruptive, you'll want to spend more time on this. Make sure everyone has access to a copy or it is visible on a computer screen and to mention each rule. In more difficult situations involving toxic behaviors, I strongly recommend that you work closely with an internal or external organizational development consultant or supportive leader to develop an effective strategy for introducing Medical Improv as culture-change tool.

   Such situations may require an organizational assessment to discover major issues involving disruptive informal power dynamics, broken trust, and/or a prevalence of bullying behaviors. Depending on how severe these problems are, consulting recommendations are likely to include leadership development,

---

[28] Jari Holland Buck, *Hospital Stay Handbook: A Guide to Becoming a Patient Advocate for Your Loved Ones,* Author-House Bloomingdale, Indiana, 2007, © by Jari Holland Buck, 2005.

specifically-designed communication training for teams, individual coaching, and possibly disciplinary actions. An organizational development consultant and/or visionary leader can help integrate the use of Medical Improv into these strategies to ensure the most positive and effective outcomes. Doing so will help prevent sabotage such as team members using informal power by refusing to cooperate, creating scheduling nightmares, or using sarcasm during play!

I also offer this special note to applied improvisers who may unwittingly become involved with toxic cultures or personalities and that is to make sure you have a champion from the organization or consider co-facilitating your workshop with a healthcare professional who understands the pressures that nurses and others face. As a nurse with over 30 years of practice, I know that healthcare professionals are up against tremendous pressures because I have been in the trenches. This gives me a credibility that allows me to nudge the group in areas like commitment to change and stretching out of their comfort zones in ways that non-healthcare professionals may not be able to do. Especially when resistance to change exists!

3. *Engage in a low-risk activity as soon as possible.* One of the best ways to help people relax is to have them experience an activity that is low risk and simple as soon as possible. *I am* is an activity you can teach before you even teach the rules. *"Yes and', 'Yes, but..."*, or *Same-Time Story* are great to introduce after a brief overview of them. These will be shared in Chapter Six.

4. *Consider a brief brainstorming session.* I often include a few brainstorming questions early in my workshops that are geared towards the skills and goals we're working on. It helps to get people engaged and talking. I've found that from the standpoint of creating a safe environment brainstorming will be more important for staff having their first experience with Medical Improv.

Make sure you review brainstorming rules, i.e. all ideas are welcome, there should be no criticizing, and ensure that everyone has a chance to offer ideas. You can do this by saying, *Let's hear from some of you who haven't shared* and/or asking people to raise hands before speaking. It is also helpful to have someone jot down responses to questions where everyone can see them i.e. on a whiteboard or poster paper. People find this validating. In larger groups I ask for tech support so that someone keys in responses that show up on a PowerPoint slide. I'll share some examples of questions and additional rationale for brainstorming in Chapter Five.

5. *Be honest and ask for support!* If this is your first time teaching this kind of activity and you trust your group, let them know that they'll be helping you practice. Unless you are dealing with toxic issues as mentioned earlier, it is fine to acknowledge that you are learning how to teach in a new way and develop your own interactive skills. I often mention that I still take improv classes and am still learning to be more assertive and many other things. You will build your own confidence by practicing with a group of colleagues who you feel confident will help make your session a positive experience. People will perceive your confidence and this will help them feel safe. Conversely, in a toxic culture, people may take advantage of your inexperience and create barriers to successful outcomes.

6. *Honor your own safety.* If you are concerned that there may be a toxic culture or any of the participants have a history of bullying or blaming behaviors consider getting a leader higher up in the hierarchy to help co-facilitate. This is a sticky area because while Medical Improv can be healing to relationships and organizational cultures, getting it off the ground in a hostile environment may backfire. Someone snickering, refusing to play, or playing with an aggressive mindset can make the experience uncomfortable or worse for everyone.

The benefit of having someone with more authority present will help ensure that staff are on their best behaviors. Even if everyone is a little more reserved, the risk of inappropriate behavior will go down while the opportunities for positive learning will still be strong. Once people get engaged in the fun and benefits, any people who might try to undermine the group's and your success will have less informal power to do so because of a growing wave of positive energy.

If you find yourself in a situation where one or more participants are being disruptive or you are perceiving them to be, I suggest calling them on it with ownership! A simple statement while looking directly at the offenders like, "I sure would appreciate respectful listening" or "Let's remember the norms we discussed" may be all it takes. If not, consider inviting disrupters to leave or voice their concerns to everyone. It is a difficult balance to hold people accountable, avoid too much time disciplining, and always role-modeling respect. Remember that your safety as well as the rest of the group's is extremely important.

7. *Be clear about expectations*. Let everyone know that different people will be learning different things, face different challenges, and that you expect everyone to be respectful. Explain that you hope people will be willing to stretch out of their comfort zones and you will encourage this, but you will never force anyone. This tip can be a great segue into spending a moment reviewing the handout and moving fairly quickly into an activity.

Using a Handout

As mentioned earlier, Medical Improv training is different from more traditional and intellectual teaching. We create the learning environment and teach the activities while the activities and participants are teaching the skills. Part of the magic with improv is that people who are participating in the same activity are learning and teaching each other different skills. As an instructor your role is more about letting this happen rather than making it happen.

For my Medical Improv workshops I create a short handout that includes these features:

- A list of possible emotional intelligence and communication skills that people might learn.
- Any session goals, objectives, or areas of impact that skill-building might help, such as: patient safety, patient experience, job satisfaction, and efficient use of resources.
- A list of core principles of Medical Improv.
- A personal action plan.

This can fit on 2 pages and is packed with information that can be used to reinforce and inspire learning that varies among individuals, arises from different activities, and continues after your session.

You will find a sample handout I used at Rutgers Medical School and a template for creating your own here:

http://www.confidentvoices.com/medical-improv-sample-handout/.

(The password, **MIPrimer2017** is intended for purchasers of this book only.)

Closing your session

As you finish a Medical Improv session I highly recommend saving a couple of minutes to debrief. During this time you can ask participants to share highlights of what they learned and how they can use the skills. If you are teaching multiple activities you can ask these questions after each one or following several activities. I also encourage a couple of minutes for quiet reflection and completing the personal action plan like this which you'll also see on the sample handouts.

Personal Action Plan

Consider today's experiences and list of skills to describe the following:

1. A strength you have in communication and collaboration.

2. One step you can take this week to use it more in your work.

3. A related skill or capacity you'd like to develop.

4. One step you can take this week to develop it in your work.

If you have more time for discussion, by all means encourage it. And don't be afraid to use this same handout repeatedly. You'll be planting seeds of awareness and learning that will continue long after your session.

As promised earlier in this chapter, *Ground Rules* provided by Jari Holland Buck, MA follow. In the next chapter we'll take some final steps to prepare you for teaching with some additional teaching strategies and resources you can use.

GROUND RULES ©
Author; Jari Holland Buck

- **CONFIDENTIALITY** — Do not talk outside of this training about specific information disclosed by other group members.
- **RISK TAKING** — Push yourself; self-disclose your ideas and feelings. By increasing risk taking, trust increases with your classmates. Risking yields trust.
- **TRUST** — Assume that no one will take action purposely intended to hurt another, so hold back no information that others could use.
- **TAKE RESPONSIBILITY/OWNERSHIP FOR LEARNING** — Come to the training prepared to learn what you need to know. That means not expecting others to feed you information and taking care of your needs (i.e., knowing when you need a break or if something is unclear).
- **LISTEN** — One person speaks at a time.
- **OK TO DISAGREE** — Everyone does not have to buy into everything said. It is preferable to have a discussion than to ignore or discount the ideas of others.
- **MUTUAL RESPECT** — Even if you do not agree, everyone needs to show respect for others. Assume class participants are competent and smart. Avoid "Zingers".
- **"I" STATEMENTS** — Speak for yourself; don't speak for others. Own your own biases.
- **GIVE/RECEIVE FEEDBACK** — The purpose of training is growth and development. If there is specific feedback you want, ask for it. Consider sharing your perceptions if they would help someone grow or would increase their self-awareness.
- **OPENNESS** — Maintain an open mind to learn new ideas. Seek to appreciate others' points of view.
- **TIMELINESS** — Please honor agreed upon schedules for breaks. If you are going to be late or need to leave early, let the group know.
- **IDEAS AREN'T BAD, QUESTIONS AREN'T STUPID** — Be an active participant and invest yourself without concern for an adverse reaction from others.
- **PARTICIPATION** — Get involved and become part of the training, sharing, and questioning.
- **HAVE FUN — ENJOY YOURSELF!**

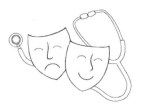

Chapter Five: Teaching Strategies & Additional Resources

In the previous chapters, we discussed the value Medical Improv can bring in addressing the challenges you face as a healthcare leader and provide you with a foundation for teaching experiential activities to improve communication and team collaboration.

In this chapter, I would like to share some additional teaching strategies and resources to help make the program a valuable tool and meet the professional development needs of your team. In this chapter we will consider the use of objectives to meet continuing education requirements, take a deeper dive into the value of brainstorming and use of a handout, and review helpful resources for continuing your own learning.

Program Objectives

Over the last decade I have customized interactive workshops for healthcare clients to meet a variety of organizational goals. The skills are typically related to emotional intelligence, communication, collaboration, and leadership. The outcomes we strive to achieve are often related to patient safety, patient experience, career satisfaction, and organizational culture.

Activities can be used or modified to emphasize different skills and contribute to a variety of goals while the objectives you use will help to help frame the learning. For instance, if I am learning to become a better listener, I will be contributing to improved patient safety, patient experience, organizational culture, and collaboration. This holds true whether you use objectives to build a workshop for continuing education credits or more informally guide the learning.

When I develop a presentation I often work with nurse educators and other healthcare leaders to develop objectives to meet the needs of the audience and to ensure the goals meet the criteria for continuing education credits. In the password-protected handout link mentioned in Chapter Four, you'll also find a list of objectives that I have successfully used and some additional ones prepared for this book. There are many ways to tweak them for your staff and organizational needs. For instance, the objective: "Describe the core principles of Medical Improv and their application to patient safety" could be easily tweaked to: "Describe the core principles of Medical Improv and their application to patient experience". Some or all of the same activities might be introduced and the teaching of the core principles will be the same, but your brainstorming questions and facilitated discussion will guide learning related to patient experience rather than patient safety. Another example of changing the learning focus using an objective from Appendix B would be to change; "Apply improved listening to ensure that patients feel heard and respected" to "Apply improved listening to ensure that staff feel heard and respected".

Because the underlying skills you are building impact everything, the objectives can vary with priorities while you enjoy knowing that the learnings will still ripple out into other areas in immeasurable ways!

While the list of objectives is presented in six categories: patient safety, patient experience, career satisfaction, organizational culture, skill-building, and teaching, there is plenty of opportunity to be creative. You might develop objectives around decreasing stress, improving morale, building positive relationships, and leadership. You might also try to test out the possibilities around optimizing resources. It's also okay, in my opinion, to do a little improv just because it is fun! Once you have your objectives you can use them to form some warm-up brainstorming questions.

Brainstorming

As mentioned in Chapter Four, a short brainstorming session can help create a safe environment and, as mentioned above, you can use your objectives to help design questions. I've developed a special format for questions that ask participants what they already know about the skill or skills, why they are important to the objectives, what the challenges or barriers are, and finally, to engage participants in the work ahead. For instance in a workshop called, *Medical Improv for Improving Communication and Collaboration among Healthcare Professionals* I would include an objective; "Explain how the core principles of Medical Improv are useful in improving assertiveness and listening". The title of the workshop and this objective can help to frame a series of brainstorming questions such as:

a. What does effective communication look like in healthcare?
b. Why is effective communication important in healthcare?
c. What are some of the challenges or barriers we face in practicing effective communication healthcare settings?
d. Are you willing to do try Medical Improv as a new way to improve communication even though there are challenges and barriers?

There are four benefits to designing questions in the above format. **First**, you'll demonstrate that for the most part everyone in the room already knows what effective communication is and why it is important. I often mention at the end of a brainstorming session that the group is obviously knowledgeable about the intellectual aspects of communication skills and that Medical Improv is a strategy that will help professionals practice them. **Second,** you'll engage participants by showing them that you are listening and making room for everyone to be heard. Many become curious when they realize this way of learning about communication honors what they know and will be different from watching another Webinar or listening to a lecture. **Third,** by asking questions that relate to the skills and goals, you'll help individuals become aware and connected to learning that is most important to them. **Fourth,** by acknowledging the challenges and barriers you'll be showing the group that you want to be honest about the realities they are facing. This may be a new and hopeful experience for many in the field and will build trust in you as a facilitator. This gives you the credibility you need to ask for cooperation from the group via the last question. It is a way of acknowledging the elephant(s) in the room and can make a big difference in the group's willingness to commit to trying Medical Improv and trust in your leadership.

As helpful as brainstorming sessions can be, they are not necessary every time you teach an activity. With experience you will become adept at employing them when it is most beneficial and when you have time. You'll also be able to advocate for time as you weigh the benefits and see the results within the context of your organization's needs.

The Handout

When I do workshops for organizations, like Rutgers Medical School, I customize a short handout to include, skills, outcomes, core principles, and a personal action plan. This becomes a tool that you can use to ask questions and participants can use to answer them. If you have a brainstorming session, it can help stimulate ideas and discussion points for learning. It can also give the audience answers to questions making it totally safe for them to think about or mention. This may seem like you are giving information away, but remember this kind of work is not about memorizing the skills. It is about raising awareness and changing individual and organizational behaviors to foster best outcomes. If one person who is generally quiet during a group discussion speaks up during brainstorming because it is safer to do so, not only does that person have the new experience of being more assertive, but everyone else has the new experience of listening and valuing that person's input. It can be a transformative moment because the next time it will be easier and a step forward in new ways of being together. Best of all, you don't have to say anything, just trust this is part of what is happening in this realm of individual and team learning.

Another benefit to keep in mind is that since participants are developing different skills, the wide range listed on the handout empowers them to identify their own strengths and opportunities for growth. In this same vein, because different participants have different experiences with the skills and outcomes, the handout can help them connect with their own stories. The learning is more memorable and you can reinforce the possibilities with debriefing questions i.e. *Reviewing the handout, did the activity help you grow in any particular areas?* Or *How might practicing this activity be helpful to us in healthcare?*

Another advantage for using a handout is that it provides another learning opportunity for those who prefer reading about the material privately or have wandering eyes while an activity or debriefing is going on. Even if they don't find me or the activity engaging, the handout might plant a seed that will contribute to the development of their emotional intelligence or communication skills over time. Some will keep the handout and find it sparks new awarenesses or reflections as in my *One Minute Death* story.

Depending on your preferences, staff, and organizational needs you might decide to narrow down the list of skill options to focus more on one area such as: listening or assertiveness. This is totally fine! And, there is one more way to use the information on the handout and that is to find out if the session was helpful.

Feedback

When I am working with a healthcare provider or conference committee to customize a presentation, one or more nurse educators, research designers, and administrators work with me to ensure organizational needs are addressed and educational criteria are met. They develop their own evaluation forms, distribute and collect completed ones, and eventually share the results with me. In addition to meeting their needs, this process is important for evaluating and improving my own teaching skills and demonstrating the usefulness of the work.

Most healthcare professionals are by necessity lifelong learners and know how objectives are used to measure the effectiveness of a workshop. For those who may not, this example will help. Take for example the **objective**: 'Demonstrate increased ability to practice assertiveness' becomes an **evaluation question**: 'To what degree are you able to demonstrate an increased ability to practice assertiveness?' The evaluation allows participants to check off the options: 'Not at all', 'Slightly', 'Moderately', 'Very', 'Extremely', or 'Not applicable'.

When I do private workshops for nurses and other healthcare professionals I ask for feedback in one or both of the following ways. First I invite verbal feedback from the group by asking, *What did you like or what was helpful?* And *What ideas do you have for making this kind of workshop better?* Here I have another chance to role model listening and if I've done a good job creating a safe environment participants will feel comfortable giving me constructive feedback and I can role-model receiving it. I may or may not write it down on a whiteboard, depending on time.

Another way to obtain relevant feedback is to create another form using the skills and outcomes listed on the sample handout or one you've created. You can add a heading and verbally ask participants to take a minute to check any skills they developed a little and circle any they developed a lot. You can use the same strategy for areas of impact or outcomes i.e. check those that were impacted a little and circle those that were impacted a lot. This method allows me to gather helpful feedback, develop the work, and provide meaningful results to my clients. And, believe it or not, it provides yet another opportunity to reinforce awareness and learning associated with all of these essential skills and critical outcomes.

As you can see, your role in teaching is not so much about presenting information as it is about creating opportunities for individual, team, and organizational learning. With Medical Improv you are always weaving in the needs of all of these along with the readiness and commitment to develop and apply skills.

Since this Primer is meant to prepare you for teaching fundamental activities, you can jump to Part III if you are itching to get started. However, it is also intended to prepare you to use other resources that are available to reinforce and further develop your teaching opportunities. The more you learn about improvisation and applied improv, the more you'll have at your fingertips to adapt for Medical Improv. Coming up are a few research oriented articles specific to Medical Improv and lots of other resources that you might find helpful in meeting your needs and those of your organization.

Resources

Over the years I've used a variety of books, articles, podcasts, and videos about improv, applied improv, and more recently Medical Improv for my own continuing education and professional development. I've also created a few of these too! What follows are brief reviews of the most helpful resources I've used. I have separated them into four categories: *philosophy/ education, academic/ research, activities/ games,* and *miscellaneous.* There is lots of overlap and many additional that I don't know about. It is my hope that this list will give you a place to start and allow you to add your own resources as you move forward in the area of Medical Improv.

Philosophy/education

Impro: Improvisation and the Theatre, by Keith Johnstone.

> Originally written in 1981 and reprinted multiple times, Johnstone's book is a fascinating look at human behavior and improvisation. His chapter on 'Status' alone is worth reading in considering the human dynamics of interprofessional and therapeutic relationships.

Theatre Games for the Classroom: A Handbook for Teachers, by Viola Spolin.

> This author is well known for her pioneering work in bridging improvisational work with social and emotional learning. This book is written for teachers who do not have a background in theatre and is geared toward elementary school-

age children. It is full of activities, many of which can be adapted for adults and her frequent examples of 'side-coaching' are invaluable. You'll also find some supportive videos and other materials at https://spolingamesonline.org/ created by well-known actor, director, and improv teacher, Gary Schwartz who studied with Spolin!

"Improvisation as a Spiritual Practice: A Deepening Path." *YouTube*, uploaded by Ted DesMaisons.

> Inspiring talk about how improv can help us grow as human beings and impact the world in positive ways.

Free Play: The Power of Improvisation in Life and the Arts by Stephen Nachmanovitch.

> Written by a musician, this is a great book for looking deeper into inspiration, creativity, and play in human beings.

Academic/research

"Improv to Improve Interprofessional Communication, Teamwork, Patient Safety, and Patient Satisfaction," Candace Campbell, 2014. A Finals Paper Project, University of San Francisco DNP program.

> Dr. Campbell's thesis is an excellent resource for evidence-based research that supports value of applied improvisational activities in helping nurses develop communication skills.

"Medical Improv: Learning Experiences that Promote Safe Care, Patient Satisfaction, & Rewarding Careers." *YouTube,* by Beth Boynton, Stephanie Frederick, and Judy White and featuring a panel of applied and medical improvisers (Lauren Dowden, Stephanie Draus, Dan Sipp, Nancy Smithner, Rich Snyder, Tobias Squier-Roper).

> This is a full length grassroots video that includes evidenced-based reasoning for Medical Improv and some fun demonstrations in the last 40 minutes.

"Perspective: Serious Play: Teaching Medical Skills With Improvisational Theater

Techniques," Professor Katie Watson, JD Academic Medicine: October 2011.

> Mentioned in Chapter One, Professor Watson's article offers evidence that improvisational activities with medical students helps them become better leaders and communicators.

"Improvisational Exercises to Improve Pharmacy Students' Professionals Communication Skills," Kevin P. Boesen, PharmD, Richard N. Herrier, PharmD, David A. Apgar, PharmD and Rebekah M. Jackowski. American Journal of Pharmaceutical Education. April, 2009.

> Ground-breaking article shows evidence that Improvisational exercises are an effective way to teach communication skills to pharmacy students.

Lifestage.org

> This website will link you to multiple resources by Jude Treder-Wolff, a social worker, educator, performer and musician. I've found her writing and resources exceptionally helpful in bridging the art and science of applied improvisation. She also offers fantastic workshops in the New York City area and I thoroughly enjoyed one called: *Connect, Communicate, & Innovate: The Improviser's Mindset in Learning & Change*. (Social Workers can obtain continuing education credits.)

Activities/games

"Applying Medical Improv in Healthcare Communication: Shifting 'Yes, But' to 'Yes, And.'" *YouTube,* uploaded by Stephanie Frederick, M.Ed, RN, and Liz Barta,

> These nurse and Medical Improv colleagues have done a fabulous job providing a three minute YouTube that demonstrates the "Yes and" core principle!

175 Theatre Games: Warm-Up Exercises for Actors by Nancy Hurley.
A great little book that separates theatre activities based on chapters like 'Teamwork and Cooperation', 'Focus and Concentration', and 'Improvisation'. There are many simple and quick activities that don't require advanced improv experience and can be useful even if not technically improv!!

Training to Imagine: Practical Improvisational Theatre Techniques for Trainers and Managers to Enhance Creativity, Teamwork, Leadership, and Learning, by Kat Koppett.

You'll find the principles of improv described differently, but don't be deterred. Add your knowledge about Medical Improv and you'll be able to use her book to add many more activities to your teaching repertoire.

ImprovEncyclopedia.org

> This website offers a comprehensive list of activities that are categorized and free to access. You'll also find a glossary and FAQ too!

ImprovDoc.org

> Dr. Belinda Fu shares some quick examples of activities at her website that help build important skills in medical students and physicians in this video on her landing page. You'll find some additional activities if you look under *concepts* and then *exercises*.

Miscellaneous

"Medline: Voices in Healthcare" *Confident Voices,*-Boynton

> I write guest posts about Medical Improv and related issues here. And try to keep a current list of podcasts, videos, and articles by myself and colleagues on my website page: www.confidentvoices.com/med-improv/.

StephanieFrederick.com (See Tab: Improv to Improv(e) Healthcare)

> Lots of great information about Medical Improv training sessions and another perspective on the principles. And do not miss the YouTube about "Yes, And" vs "Yes, But"!

MedicalImprov.org: Professor Katie Watson and Dr. Belinda Fu's website.

> If you are interested in attending their Train-the-Trainer program you'll find

information there as well as more about them and all of the Alum!

Applied Improvisation Network

You can find the website (http://appliedimprovisation.network/) and Facebook page (https://www.facebook.com/groups/appliedimprov/) for this active and growing group. There are lots of podcasts, a small Medical Improv subgroup; regional groups that meet in-person, ongoing events, and lots of resources. I try to attend meetings of the Applied Improv Network New England!

Of course you'll find lots more online and these links will lead you to others. Maybe your community offers an improv course that is or isn't geared towards actors. In the meantime, let's move on to the final chapters on fundamental improv activities that you are now ready to facilitate with your staff, colleagues, teams, and organizations!

Part III: 15 Fundamental Activities You Can Teach STAT!

Now you are ready to teach fundamental Medical Improv activities and help healthcare professionals provide safer care and ensure optimal patient experience while finding more joy and meaning in their work. The potential rippling effects into teams, organizations, the healthcare system, and society at large could be immeasurable!

The activities are listed in three categories: Emotional Intelligence and Communication, Teamwork, & Leadership and Followership. Each set is arranged in order of slightly increasing risk and complexity and there is a general increase in both with activities in Chapters Seven and Eight. In addition to describing the activity and offering sample scenarios, we will look at estimates on time needed, skills to emphasize, facilitation tips, debriefing questions, and variations to consider. There is also a space for you to write notes about what worked best or new ideas as I am sure you will have some.

Please know that I am making every effort to cite resources I've used for original material, but there are several with unknown sources. Many activities are well known, commonly practiced, and handed down and modified from improv group to improv group, but their origins are not clearly documented.

If you have questions or feedback, please write to me at beth@bethboynton.com.

PART THREE

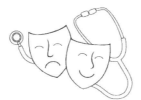

Chapter Six: 5 Activities for Improving Emotional Intelligence & Communication

Activity # 1: *I am* (Source unknown)

Purpose: This exercise is in writing and at its deepest roots creates space for awareness and respect of self and others which are fundamental to emotional intelligence and communication. By making time for *I am* you will be giving staff the message that each and every one is important and that is is okay to focus on self and others outside the clinical realm for a few minutes.

Healthcare professionals have generally been encouraged to take care of patients, but not themselves. This contributes to a mixed message about speaking up and contributes to errors associated with fatigue, stress, and feeling rushed. As simple as *I am* is, it helps to create the psychological safety necessary to acknowledge and set healthy limits, speak up about patient concerns, give and receive constructive feedback, share ideas about quality improvement, and respect needs of others, even when they are different from one's own. Believe it or not, this simple activity can even help address safe staffing by setting the stage for accepting our own and each other's limits!

It is also simple and fun way for people to get to know and appreciate each other!

Time needed: 10 minutes

Skills: The very essence of *I am* promotes self-awareness, self-reflection, self-respect, and respect for others. It builds trust and promotes empathy and positive relationships as people take a few minutes to get to know what is important to each other and discover what they have in common or be surprised by differences.

Description: Have staff write down (or include in your handout): *I am* _____ three times on a piece of paper. Then ask them to fill in the blanks with three things about themselves they are willing to share with 2-3 others in the group. I usually give examples such as;

> *I am excited to meet with you today.*
>
> *I am stressed about the new EMR we have.*
>
> *I am going on vacation after this workshop.*

Allow a couple of minutes to complete and then ask the group to exchange *I ams* with others for about 5 min. I encourage all the participants to walk around the room spending a minute or so with each of 2-3 people. This way each person will share their *I ams* with and learn about 2-3 others. Make sure to let people know they will be sharing their *I ams* with others and they should only write down things they feel comfortable sharing.

Facilitation: Encourage participants to spend equal time sharing their own and reading each other's *I ams*. Typically *I am* starts out very quiet, and I have to remind myself to let that be. After a minute or two, the conversations start and soon the room gets noisy as participants begin talking with and listening to each other! As with all activities, make sure you have explained a process for letting them loose and reeling them back in as discussed in Chapter Four.

You do not need to teach the rules of Medical Improv prior to doing this activity and it can be used as a warmup to engage participants with other work and each other. Some participants may feel *I am* is a frivolous use of time and/or have some discomfort in sharing or learning about others. Keep in mind that for some people either may be a new experience. After validating concerns, reassure them that it is is a very powerful activity that builds relationships, emotional intelligence and communication.

Debriefing: You and your staff might be surprised at how the energy shifts in a positive direction as people engage and connect with each other. I often walk away thinking that people are indeed starving for healthy interactive time that is not clinically oriented. And as facilitators, we provide a structure that empowers people to do what they are naturally inclined to do; care about each other!

Some questions you can use to spark discussion and reinforce experiential learning:

- What did you notice about this activity?
- How might this activity can be connected to assertiveness, listening, emotional intelligence and/or other growth?
- Which was more comfortable, sharing with or learning about others?
- How is this activity helpful or useful to the unit?
- Did anyone find it challenging and, if so, are they willing to say more?

Variations: This activity can be used more than once with the same group and different mixes of staff. It can be extremely helpful in breaking down tension or silos between shifts or departments. Depending on group mix and how much relationship building you want to promote, encourage sharing with at least one person they don't know too well. *I am* can be tweaked to focus on a particular organizational initiative or topic, e.g. advise them to complete their sentences with respect to creating a culture of safety or improving patient experience.

Notes:

Activity # 2: *Yes and…, Yes but…., and No!* (Adapted from Keith Johnstone's Impro: Improvisation and the Theatre.)

Purpose: This verbal activity teaches the Yes and principle of Medical Improv while giving participants insights into how it feels to support each other and be supported. It also helps to raise awareness about one's own behavior in resisting, contradicting, or not listening to others with an open mind and promotes collaborative communication among doctors and nurses, nurses and nurses, clinicians and patients, administrators and staff. There is a great and brief video[29] by colleagues Stephanie Frederick, M.Ed, RN and Liz Barta, RN, BSN, CHES that demonstrates how practicing this activity can lead to more collaborative conversations. It's called, "Applying Medical Improv in Healthcare Communication. Shifting 'Yes, But' to 'Yes, And'"!

Time needed: 15-20 minutes

Skills: Both assertiveness and listening are key. They both also raise awareness about taking or not taking risk, feeling or not feeling validated, and the overall tone of collaboration.

Description: To teach this three-part activity, the group breaks up into pairs taking on the numbers 1 and 2. The pairs are instructed to have a conversation about a general topic, such as sports, pets, vacations, etc. They must alternate one sentence at a time and with the exception of the very first one, all sentences must begin with *Yes and….* Ask them to go back and forth 3 or 4 times so that each person comes up with 3 or 4 sentences. Give them an example such as with the topic of pets:

> **Person 1:** *I am going to get a new puppy today.*
>
> **Person 2:** *Yes, and you sound very excited about this new family member.*
>
> **Person 1:** *Yes, and my son has already named the puppy, Pokeman!*

Allow for a couple of minutes for pairs to work together and then reel them back in. You

---

[29] Stephanie Frederick and Liz Barta, "Applying 'Medical' Improv in Healthcare Communication: Shifting 'Yes, But' to 'Yes, And,'" *YouTube*, upload August 10, 2015, https://www.YouTube.com/watch?v=riseDHKLgP8.

don't need to do much debriefing at this juncture although it can be helpful to invite general feedback about the experience. Next, and in the same pairs, ask participants to have a conversation about a different topic where they alternate one sentence at a time 3-4 times as before. This time and with the exception of the very first one, all sentences must begin with *Yes, but...*

> **Person 1**: *I am going to pack my suitcase for our trip to New York City.*
>
> **Person 2**: *Yes, but I loaned your suitcase to my sister.*
>
> **Person 1**: *Yes, but, I borrowed one from my friend.*

This conversation doesn't have to continue for very long before participants realize how defensive and uncooperative they are being together. Conversations like these typically don't go very far. In a safe and low-risk way, they gain awareness of how if feels, looks, and sounds like to have a conversation with a colleague that is not very supportive.

Feedback and debriefing can take place at this point or followed by one more quick conversation where participants answer each other with *No*, e.g.:

> **Person 1**: *I am going join a bowling team this winter.*
>
> **Person 2**: *No. The bowling alley burned down last week.*

Facilitation: This activity can be used to introduce or reinforce the core principle of Medical Improv because the profound experiences of contrast drives home the point of *Yes and!* Choose and vary topics that are safe to talk about and that most people can relate to. Some examples include: yard work, social media, cooking, or continuing education! Remind them that they can make things up.

It is worth mentioning that some participants like to make the point that we can't always agree in healthcare and that disagreeing can be a life-saving intervention. This is true! When it comes up in discussion or if you decide to bring it up yourself, you can speak to the difference between Medical Improv vs. real work situations. In Medical Improv we're developing skills to improve our overall communication and collaboration whereas in healthcare we're collaborating for optimal outcomes such as patient experience and safety. In the clinical arena, dissenting opinions take on a different and very essential role, yet ensuring all voices are heard, still requires practice in listening and speaking up. Learning and practicing *Yes and* helps to create a foundation for the skill and psychological safety necessary to speak up and be heard when a *Yes, but* is necessary!

Debriefing: As this activity unfolds in real time, participants might be experiencing some profound and possibly painful awarenesses about their tendency to invalidate others and/or how it feels to be invalidated and, in either case, what this can do to the tone of a conversation. As you facilitate discussion on this learning be sure to keep psychological safety in mind and invite, but never push disclosure. For some people, the awarenesses will continue to evolve long after your session is over. I often receive feedback from people days or weeks after a workshop saying, "I just had a *Yes and* conversation instead of a *Yes, but!*" It exemplifies the power of experiential learning and the rippling effect it can have on our communication, collaboration, and culture.

Some questions you can use to spark discussion and reinforce experiential learning:

- What did you notice about this activity?
- How did the quality of conversations differ?
- How did the different conversations make you feel?
- How can you use *Yes and* even when you don't agree?
- How might this activity be helpful in clinical or administrative meetings?

Variations: It is ok to skip the third conversation with *No,* although it can be useful in experiencing what it is like to be denied. This notion makes it a useful leadership activity in terms of building empathy for staff or others who may have limited choices. If time is limited, you can have two people demonstrate *Yes and* and *Yes but* conversations while facilitating discussion among the group.

Notes:

Activity # 3: *Same-time story aka Mirror Speech aka Synchronized Story* (Adapted from Viola Spolin's Theater for the Classroom.)

Purpose: This activity builds attentive listening skills by creating an opportunity for people to focus entirely on someone else. As clinicians our listening is often limited to asking questions and checking off boxes. In this activity participants get to experience a deep sense of feeling heard and practice the kind of listening that transcends assessment. It is important to cultivate the ability to listen in this way and it is quite different! Here we stop thinking of the million other things we need to do or problems we have at home and listen to understand others and show that we care about them.

While we may not always have time to focus this intently on any one patient or colleague, (a sad reality for many and one that I don't condone) the activity can be extremely helpful for increasing ability to recognize when this kind of listening is most important and how to do it. For example, a patient who is expressing anxiety in the middle of the night about upcoming surgery or a colleague who seems to be on the verge of tears as the shift begins signal times when putting down our pens and paper or computer screen and simply listening is the priority.

Intuitively, we can imagine that the trust and emotional safety experienced will engage and empower others in immeasurable ways. For example, consider how knowing that your colleagues care about you could impact bullying behaviors on the unit or how a patient feeling cared for by the healthcare team could influence a surgical outcome!

Time needed: 15 minutes

Skills: Listening and emotional intelligence concepts, including identifying social cues, increasing trust, and developing empathy.

Description: In this activity pairs of participants face each other and take turns telling a story with their partner at the same time. One person acts as the storyteller while the other tries to say exactly what their partner is saying at the same time. Each turn should last a minute or so and there should be a pause and change of topics between turns. Have the storyteller start with a phrase such as *One day I was...* or *Once upon a time I....* This prompt helps the storyteller get started and helps the follower know what the first few words will be so they can start to get in sync. In order to do this the storyteller must go slowly and the story mirrorer must pay close attention to what their partner is saying or going to say.

Also, you can provide optional story topics such as *the day you won a million dollars*, *the time you caught a Great White shark*, or *the mysterious gift you received from your grandmother*. Allow a minute to decide topic and if participants want to make up or tell a true story, that is fine!

Facilitation: This can be a confusing activity to explain, yet easy to understand when demonstrated, and the debriefing is well worth the effort. I either coach two people in a trial or have someone demonstrate with me. In the latter, it can be more helpful if you are the storyteller so you can go at a slow enough pace that your follower can be successful. Once participants engage in the activity, walk around the room and listen to pairs so you can gently remind them to slow down, support their partner, and that it is okay to make things up.

Debriefing: Some of the exciting feedback that you might get with this activity might be participants who share that they've *never felt heard like this before* or *been so attuned to another person*. Some questions you can use to spark discussion and reinforce experiential learning:

- What did you notice about the activity?
- Was either telling the story or mirroring easier or more comfortable?
- What were you thinking about when you were mirroring? (Usually people are not focusing on anything else besides what their partner is saying and this is a great point to highlight.)
- Any comments from storytellers about feeling heard? (Another great point to highlight.)
- How can you use the learning in your clinical or other workplace setting? (I often mention that while this kind of listening may not feel realistic all the time, it can be a helpful approach to use when a patient, colleague, or employee seem anxious or overwhelmed or appear to be getting angry. Such situations can signal a time to use the kind of focused or attentive listening skills developed in this activity.)

It is also worth mentioning that I received a complaint once that the activity "...felt like it was a distraction from listening". I suspect others have felt similarly, but were not so willing to share. It was a great reminder for me that Medical Improv is not for everyone or, at the very least, more challenging for some. My sense was that this participant had a hard time giving up control while they were listening and although their listening to assess skills were astute, their ability to connect this deeply with another may have felt threatening. I validated their feedback and thanked them for it. I also asked if I could challenge them a bit and with permission asked what they felt they were being distracted from; this lead to comments about not being able to focus on the story itself. This sparked a valuable discussion about how 80-90% of our communication is nonverbal and how this activity, which involves a made up story could help participants develop awareness about what is going on between us aside from the content. The point isn't to teach ignoring content, but rather to bring into balance other important communication that is going on!

I also reminded the participant about the option to observe for the rest of the activity. They chose to continue and I hope experienced some positive growth in the moment or upon subsequent reflection.

Variations: In larger groups you can break into groups of three or four and have observers who are tasked with paying close attention to anything related to emotional intelligence, communication or collaboration. Break this up into a two-part activity where in one meeting two people demonstrate for a longer period while the rest of the group observes. In a subsequent meeting have people break into pairs and do the activity. You can also get story ideas from the group. Even if the debriefing is a little repetitive that is ok because the experiential learning will be different. Since this activity also helps to form more trusting relationships, you can be intentional about pairing up staff that may have some tension between them. It is a judgment call and likely to be helpful with mild to moderate conflict and less so with major or old hostility. Be mindful of doing this after people are more comfortable with the activity.

CHAPTER SIX

Notes:

Activity # 4: *Accept This!* (Adapted from Kat Koppett's, *Training to Imagine*.)

Purpose: This activity helps reinforce the *Yes and* core principle of Medical Improv while creating opportunities to see others express a variety of emotions and try them out. Because some people are more comfortable expressing some emotions while uncomfortable with others, this activity provides a safe way to practice.

Accept this builds skills that are associated with recognizing emotional tones in others and developing one's own abilities to be aware of and express feelings. This can be helpful in a variety of clinical situations where early recognition of escalating anger or depression would be helpful in shifting one's approach to listening, determining clinical priorities, and guide appropriate interventions. It is also helpful in developing the ability to manage one's own emotions.

In addition to the principals of Medical Improv and facilitating a safe environment for taking emotional risks, this activity also makes expressing emotions safer for two additional reasons. First, because individuals are given permission to be expressive and second, because the emotional charge of reacting is minimized. In other words *Accept This* gives individuals a green light to express happy, sad, angry, or tired feelings without a major extrinsic cause which may invoke fears of judgments and inhibit one's self-expression. For instance, expressing anger has been an emotion that is challenging for me and this activity has helped me to feel a little more comfortable trying it out.

The positive rippling effect of developing such emotional intelligence can help individuals and the system become and stay healthier in a variety of ways. A doctor or nurse who can defuse anger in a patient will be less likely to be injured and more likely to build a positive relationship which may have a significant impact on a patient's willingness to trust the practitioner and comply with clinical advice. Clinicians who are in touch with their own feelings may identify and seek help for signs of burnout earlier and last a lot longer in their position, or seek a healthier job match. In any case, practitioners will be healthier and able to provide safer care!

Time needed: 20 minutes

Skills: Identifying feelings in self and others, self-expression of range of primary emotions, self-awareness of feelings, listening to others' expression of emotions, empathy.

Facilitation: As you begin to teach this activity, include an opportunity to demonstrate or ask for input about what a neutral or mundane tone would sound and look like and relate it to what we clinically describe as a flat affect. You might also have examples of mundane statements available to use or brainstorm ideas before starting.

Depending on time you can debrief between each emotion and invite input about what a 'big reaction' looks and sounds like as well as verbal and nonverbal signs of the five different emotions. Also, a word of caution here, and that is to remind participants that even with 'big reactions' everyone should be respectful. It is possible that some individuals who have repressed emotions like anger or sadness might be so liberated that their reactions border on being out of control. I've never experienced or witnessed this in an improv class, but do recall teaching a communication workshop where I had a nurse role-playing an angry surgeon and she went into a rage and got in my personal space. I put up my hands to signal her to stop and she did, but it surprised me a bit.

Debriefing: There are many examples where raising awareness of feelings could help us and your staff will probably have some great ideas about this. For example, I believe that if we all honor our own and each other's feelings a little bit more, we will have a continuous and positive impact on bullying and blaming cultures. Therefore, practicing outside our high stakes high stress work environments is a very productive use of everyone's time! As you facilitate discussion, you can certainly guide it in a direction that your unit or organization is working on, such as improving patient experience or working to eliminate a bullying culture. Some questions you can use to spark discussion and reinforce experiential learning:

- How was the experience?
- Were any of the emotions more or less comfortable for you to express?
- Were any of the emotions more or less comfortable for you to listen to?
- When is it important to identify feelings in patients and families, colleagues, ourselves?
- How can identifying feelings help us care for patients and families, colleagues, ourselves?
- What kind of differences might the above make in clinical outcomes? How about job satisfaction and performance? Other areas?

Variations: You can use pairs to demonstrate any part of this activity and facilitate larger group discussions. (Keep in mind the experiential learning for those expressing emotions may be greater.) Write the emotions down on pieces of paper and show only to the person who will be expressing each one. Then have the group observe guess what emotion it was and what made them draw that conclusion. Spread the activity over several sessions with a different emotion being focused on. You can also invite brainstorming about what emotions might be used by asking for some common feelings that patients (or colleagues) might have and then use them in the process.

Notes:

Activity # 5: *The Gift* (Adapted from Kat Koppett's, *Training to Imagine,* Professor Katie Watson's curriculum and June 2012 Train-the-Trainer program, and in subsequent and lengthy conversation with Terry Sommer and Ed Dunn, MD following the training.) Terry and I were helping Ed tweak and practice the activity so that he could use it in a new program to help prepare healthcare professionals for making apologies associated with medical errors and disclosure!

Purpose: This activity is a wonderful way to help healthcare professionals become more comfortable with sharing responsibility and power in communication and less defensive when skills or knowledge are challenged. This will be extremely helpful in promoting effective communication in many situations and at all levels.

As one person gives an invisible gift, it is the other person's responsibility to define what the gift is. In traditional improv, this activity teaches actors to co-create a scene. In Medical Improv, participants experience sharing power in a safe way and internalize understanding about the important difference between validating someone and agreeing with them. To understand the value of this activity before teaching it, here are some examples of how it can contribute to deep experiential learning and shift persistent and pervasive old patterns in new and positive directions.

Old way:

> **Staff Nurse:** *We need more nurses on this unit.*
>
> **Nurse Manager:** *We don't have the budget for any more nurses.*

New way:

> **Staff Nurse:** *We need more nurses on this unit.*
>
> **Nurse Manager:** *Sounds like you think more nurses would be helpful, yes?*

In the *old way* we have a power struggle between leader and staff nurse that contributes to disengagement of staff, separation between staff and leaders, and lack of full understanding about staffing issues and collaborative problem-solving. In the *new way* the power struggle has been avoided and the door to collaborative problem-solving is now open. As you and your staff gain awareness about this nebulous concept, you will start to see how this old pattern manifests and creates problems in many areas.

Old way:

>**Patient:** *I hate to take medications.*
>
>**Doctor:** *If you don't, there is a good chance you'll have a stroke.*

New way:

>**Patient:** *I hate to take medications.*
>
>**Doctor:** *You don't like the idea of taking medications? Tell me more.*

Old way:

>**Staff Nurse 1:** *I'm really stressed out. I don't think I can handle another admission.*
>
>**Staff Nurse 2:** *I had two admissions yesterday and was fine!*

New way:

>**Staff Nurse 1:** *I'm really stressed out. I don't think I can handle another admission.*
>
>**Staff Nurse 2:** *Sounds like you are pretty stressed. I'd help if I could. Have you talked with the Charge Nurse?*

Old way:

>**Patient:** *Ow, that hurt. Can you get someone who knows how to start an IV?*
>
>**Staff Nurse:** *Hold still. I've done hundreds of these.*

New way:

> **Patient:** *Ow, that hurt. Can you get someone who knows how to start an IV.*
>
> **Staff Nurse:** *That hurt, didn't it? I'm sorry. I'm usually pretty good at starting IVs are you ok with me trying one more time? I promise to get someone else if I'm not successful.*

As these examples suggest, validating other perspectives is a key listening skill that helps manage conflict, demonstrates respect, empowers patients and staff, and offers genuine apologies when indicated. As you will see, *The Gift* can be an important stepping stone to promoting respectful communication among all stakeholders!

Time needed: 15 minutes

Skills: Assertiveness and listening, (especially validation) are emphasized as well as sharing power, all of which are essential in collaborative work, managing conflict, and empowering others. It is helpful in identifying social cues when an emphasis is placed on observers, (see variations) and can promote creativity, flexibility, and positive relationships.

Description: In pairs participants take turns giving each other invisible gifts. They should be sitting or standing and facing each other. What each gift is will be determined by the receiver while the giver validates.

> **Person 1** hands an invisible gift to Person 2 saying something like: *Here's a present for you.*
>
> **Person 2** takes the invisible gift, tells Person 1 what it is, and adds a bit about it: *Oh thank you for my new hat. I'm going to wear it to the party tonight.*
>
> **Person 1** builds on Person 2's idea: *I thought it would go perfectly with your new coat!*

At this point person 2 should give a gift to person 1 and so on. Participants should each give each other 3 gifts in this way and depending on time, repeat with one or more new partners.

Facilitation: Keep your eyes out for people who may seem to struggle a bit with either role so that you can encourage following the rules of the activity and signal any celebrations of risk-taking for pauses or mistakes. You can also make a mental note about who might be willing to share what felt challenging during the debrief.

For example, a surgeon who is used to giving orders might find it awkward to have someone else tell her what gift she is giving while a nurse who is used to following orders might have a little trouble defining something for another. Both of these practitioners can grow in major ways by experiencing a different way of being together.

In this place or space, the surgeon is making room for the nurse's views and in doing so has the opportunity to experience being open and collaborative while showing respect for the nurse. This may be a foreign concept to a surgeon and helpful in developing rapport with the surgical team. In this same place or space, the nurse is learning to take the risk of speaking up about a concern to authority. This risk-taking in a safe way may be just as foreign to the nurse and will help build confidence and important awareness about any hesitation that might occur in any clinical communication. And not only do these professionals experience profound self-growth, they are building a respectful relationship and making surgery safer.

This dynamic, although more subtle, is present in many relationships with peers, patients, and leaders and any resistance to sharing power can be useful to reflect on.

As a facilitator it can be helpful to realize that in this space, that may be a little uncomfortable, participants are learning to take on and share more power than they are used to. It is an important part of practicing respectful communication where both or all parties have value and is extremely important in collaboration, managing conflict, giving and receiving constructive feedback, and empowering others. As such, this seemingly simple improvisational activity helps to provide a foundation for the kind of communication necessary for establishing and sustaining a culture of safety.

Debriefing: This activity is so simple that without expert facilitation profound learning can be lost. Being cognizant of the above discussion will help you to guide the debriefing towards such important learning. Try to let participants figure out the answers and provide examples when necessary. Some questions you can use to spark discussion and reinforce experiential learning:

- What did you notice about the activity?
- Was there any nonverbal communication going on? What did it seem to mean?
- Any thoughts about what might make one role more challenging than another? How could you tell?
- Which was more comfortable for you, receiving and identifying the gift or validating it?
- Can you draw any conclusions about participating in this activity in terms of communication?
- How can this activity be helpful to us in clinical or administrative situations?

Variations: Do in a circle formation with 6-10 in each circle so that the gift-giving and receiving goes is in a circular pattern where person 1 gives to person 2 and person 2 gives to person 3, etc. Repeat the pattern in the other direction. This will allow for more observations to the interactions. Another way to do this is to form groups of 4 where two people are charged with giving and receiving gifts while two observers are asked to note any nonverbal language that might be going on during the exchange.

Notes:

Now that you've helped individuals become their best selves, inspired continued growth, and introduced the concept of Medical Improv as a fun way to learn, you are ready to focus more on collaborative work or leadership and followership. There is a natural overlap in that leadership includes followership and both are essential in teamwork. Separating these out, allows for a wider variety of activities and skills that will inherently dovetail for synergistic skill development!

In the next chapter we'll focus on activities that help individuals become more effective communicators in teams while continuing to develop emotional intelligence.

CHAPTER SIX

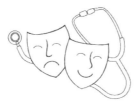

Chapter Seven: 5 Activities for Improving Teamwork

As discussed in Chapter Two, the limitations we face in practicing respectful communication and behavior are significant—taking the risks of speaking up and listening become even more complex and stressful in groups. It is common knowledge that many people are anxious or even phobic about public speaking. Fears about judgment and/or conflict help explain why. Further, fears about speaking up in a team can be hindered by blaming or bullying cultures that provide tacit yet powerful messages about perceived dangers of speaking up. Ramifications for speaking up whether real or perceived or aggressive or passive-aggressive, include job loss, humiliation, unfair workloads, and/or being ignored, overlooked, or excluded from activities. This combination of individual anxieties and toxic cultures is complex and powerful influence on patient care and career satisfaction.

It is also worth mentioning that healthcare teams and the patients they care for are more and more diverse, including differences in status and place within the organizational hierarchy, educational background, ethnicity, work experience, gender, age, and personality. Whether diversity is welcomed and trusted or resisted and feared can make a huge difference in how teams perform and the care they provide.

Medical Improv activities provide safe, fun, and healthy interactions that are like a positive counterforce. Over time and with more and more positive experiences together, individual and organizational behaviors will shift into healthier ways of working together.

The activities in this chapter provide continued development of emotional intelligence and communication skill-building in groups by balancing psychological safety and emotional risk-taking. This balance is necessary for mastering the skills, gaining confidence, building trust, and developing positive relationships in teams. All of which are essential for collaborative and safe teamwork as the minute-to-minute demands of high stakes, high stress patient care unfold.

The next five activities are designed to help healthcare professionals feel safer, be more effective communicating in groups, and help to dissolve tensions between shifts and departments.

Activity # 6: *Let's Plan a Party* (Adapted from a collaborative workshop developed with Terry Sommer for a special session teaching improv to nursing students at Mount Sinai Beth Israel, Fall 2015)

Purpose: This activity is designed to help healthcare professionals internalize what collaborative and non-collaborative teamwork looks, feels, and sounds like. This will pave the way for more supportive behaviors and continued heightened awarenesses as participants encounter many opportunities to practice at work.

If you've ever been to a meeting where a change initiative or other organizational goal is being discussed and where one or two people seem to affect the group in a negative way, you will quickly grasp how valuable this exercise can be. Typically, everyone can feel this kind of destructive power, but it is elusive and difficult to address. *Let's Plan a Party* will help your group become more aware of how people's emotional tone and behavior impacts others. This increase in awareness in the group will make it a more visible influence and with that, more accountability for respectful behavior.

Time needed: 20 min (Allow more time for larger group)

Skills: Raises awareness about respectful listening and assertiveness in teamwork and increases ability to do so. Also helpful in developing a team culture where all voices are spoken and heard and including safe space for dissenting opinions.

Description: In this activity, teams of 6-8 participants plan a party (birthday, Halloween, retirement, etc.) in two different ways. (Multiple groups can play at the same time). In the first session, they are to go around in a the circle with each person making a suggestion about planning the party while the other members of the team offer supportive responses that add a little more detail to the idea, i.e. *Yes, and…*! In the second round, each person offers a suggestion while the group responds with reasons they can think of about why it won't work or is a bad idea i.e. *Yes, but…*! Here's what it would look like with a group of six:

Round one of *Let's plan a birthday party for Betsy:*

> **Person 1:** *Let's get some decorations to put up in her office!*
>
> **Person 2:** *Great idea, her favorite color is green.*

Person 3: *She'll love it. I'll pick up some crepe paper.*

Person 4: *Excellent idea! She'll be so surprised!*

Person 5: *Perfect plan. I'll buy some balloons.*

Person 6: *Great! She'll get a big kick out of it.*

Then person 2 makes a suggestion and so forth. In Round Two, use a different party idea, such as plan a holiday party for everyone, it would look like this:

Person 1: *Let's have a holiday party after work next week!*

Person 2: *I don't think people really feel like celebrating.*

Person 3: *Let's not try to have a party after work everyone will be too tired.*

Person 4: *I'd rather find a way to have a party on a day I'm not working.*

Person 5: *You can if you want, but I don't have time to cook anything for it.*

Person 6: *I think it would be better to wait until after the holidays when everyone isn't so stressed.*

Facilitation: You can start this session with a quick brainstorm of reasons to have a party and write them down so they are visible. Leave it up to each group what parties they will plan and encourage them to plan different parties for each round so they can tap into new ideas. It is a little safer to have group size be closer to 6 because it is more intimate and require less supportive or dissenting ideas

Debriefing: As you lead the discussion, keep in mind that neither you nor the group needs to point fingers at any individuals who have a tendency to bring negative power into the group. In fact, doing so would be inappropriate and possibly shaming. Such individuals will probably be absorbing some feedback about their own behavior from the activity itself. They might grow and change with the new knowledge or perhaps there are other personnel issues that are being addressed privately. Keep the focus on positive change and forward movement and remind the group that we've all had bad days and moods!

It is worth mentioning here that individual and organizational behaviors are interrelated and complex. Although, it may be tempting to blame individuals for poor behavior like bullying and seek solutions like termination, I believe leaders must first provide feedback, clear expectations, and an opportunity to learn. *Let's Plan a Party,* while not intended to be the sole approach to any of these, does provide some of each!

Some questions you can use to spark discussion and reinforce experiential learning:

- What kinds of things did you notice about the two rounds?
- Which round felt safer to be creative?
- Does encouraging ideas mean agreeing with them?
- How can encouraging ideas help create space for dissenting opinions?
- What suggestions do you have for ensuring room for both in your team(s)?
- Is it worth spending a few minutes participating in this activity? Why or why not?

Variation: Another way to play this activity is to have the whole group participate in a big circle (this works for work for 16 or so). In this case someone starts by making a suggestion and the person to his right offers a supportive statement while the rest of the group offers supportive sounds, words, and gestures together. Then the next person to the right offers a negative response while the rest of the participants support the dissenter. Each person in the circle offers a suggestion going around clockwise.
In a big circle it would look something like this for planning a Halloween party.

> **Person 1:** *I think we should turn the staff lounge into a haunted house for Halloween.*
>
> **Person 2:** *Yes, what a great idea. We can all dress up!*
> Everyone else nods, cheers, and agrees that it is a great idea.
>
> **Person 3:** *But, that's going to make a big mess right in the middle of the day.*
> Everyone else grimaces and groans in agreement with person 3.
>
> **Person 2:** *We could have a contest for coming up with the best costume and give away movie tickets.*

Person 3: *Definitely! I can't wait to dress up.*
Everyone else nods, cheers, and agrees that it is a great idea.

Person 4: *I think it will cause a lot of tension because it is so competitive.*
Everyone else grimaces and groans in agreement with person 3.

And so on!

Notes:

Activity # 7: *The Know-it-All* also called the *Three Headed Monster* or *Ask Waldo* (Source unknown).

Purpose: This activity requires participants to rely on and be flexible with each other as they create the answer to questions together. In healthcare, there are many teams working to provide patient care, and the people who comprise any particular team will vary with the shift, staffing patterns, patient needs, skill set and experience, and other clinical and nonclinical factors. In the almost constantly changing ebbs and flows of providing care, all members of healthcare teams must be able to speak up about concerns. This also means that all members must be able to listen to concerns from any other team player at any moment!

Intellectually, this seems simple, but we know that it is not. Engaging staff and creating psychologically safe environments for speaking up are both challenges that leaders in healthcare organizations face. Although a generalization, the old hierarchy, regardless of intention, has left us with some bad habits involving nurses who don't speak up and doctors who don't listen!

Some will be challenged more by sharing an idea and others by accepting it. Consider how both involve impulses that may be connected to core human beliefs that drive behavior. For instance, I've learned a lot about my own assertiveness in improv classes because I have come to recognize what I would describe as a gut instinct to hesitate when I have an idea or concern. Now, at this point in my life, it has little to do with my actual behavior, because I am aware of it and don't let it. This gut instinct arises from my life experiences, work as a nurse, and neurological response to the risk I perceive. All of which contribute to my conviction that assertiveness is way more complicated than it appears! I remember giving my first Keynote address at the Washington Nurses Association annual conference a few years ago. At the time, I had finished my first book, completed my Master's degree, and had over 20 years of nursing when I shared a story about being more anxious about taking a clinical concern up the ladder in my direct care position than I was giving that presentation[30]!

I've come to believe that listening includes a similar challenge because, at its deepest

---

[30] Beth Boynton, "Recognizing the Complexity of Assertiveness is Key to Providing Effective Training & Promoting 'Speak Up' Behaviors Among Patients & Nurses," *Confident Voices in Healthcare*, October 5, 2012, http://tinyurl.com/hlp2g64

core, there are fears about loss of control. Listening is easier or perhaps more natural for me personally, and yet if there is a situation where I feel vulnerable, in conflict, or for any reason like I need to be in charge, it is harder to let someone else's opinion or perspective in. So I wonder, what it might feel like to a physician who has been taught to be in charge all the time, to listen to patients and nurses who also have very important expertise. Does this feel threatening in some way?

If we are willing, as teachers, to acknowledge that improving communication in healthcare teams may involve emotional risk-taking by members of the team, we can understand why our clinical environments do not support this kind of personal growth. We're too rushed and our old habits are familiar. Not safer for patients, but in some deep-rooted emotional place, safer for us.

The Know-it-All is a very useful exercise in cultivating new habits of speaking up and listening. And if you are fortunate enough to have a leadership which supports doctors and nurses working in the same workshop, the experiences can be transformative.

Time needed: 15 Minutes

Skills: Increasing confidence in speaking up and listening in small groups, coping with change, creativity. When played with peers will also build trust and improve relationships.

Description: 3 people sit side by side and answer open-ended questions from the audience going from left to right and one word at a time. The answers do not need to be factual, but do need to have a sensible flow. The audience asks these open-ended questions about the mysteries of life or anything they'd like to know about. It is helpful to have participants begin their answer by rephrasing the question and would look something like this:

> Question: *Why is the sky blue?*
>
> Nurse: *The*
>
> Nurse Manager: *sky*
>
> Surgeon: *is*

> **Nurse:** *blue*
>
> **Nurse Manager:** *because*
>
> **Surgeon:** *atmospheric*

And so forth until the sentence has been completed. The other participants can then nod and make hmmmmmms in appreciation of this important information. Allow each threesome to answer a couple of questions and then have *The Know-it-all* shift to the left so that one person leaves and another joins.

Facilitation: Coaching includes reminders of only speaking one word at a time, celebrating risk-taking, continuing to move forward when someone makes a mistake, and building a sensible response. Allow for a couple of rounds as people get the hang of it and then encourage a faster pace. Also remind participants that questions that ask for yes or no, numbers, or location responses are not open-ended.

As this activity plays out you will notice some participants thinking and planning their answers. This becomes clear when the person next to them says something that foils their plan and requires them to go in a different direction. In between each person's contribution is a rich field of listening, flexibility, critical thinking, assertiveness, and cooperation.

To make this point clearer let's go back to the above example when the surgeon said *atmospheric*. He may have had an idea about atmospheric pressure and visual physiology that might seem like the most sensible path for the story to continue, yet does not know what the nurse next in line is thinking or will say. Conversely, the nurse may be worried that what he will say will be different from what the surgeon has in mind. In this case, the nurse may be thinking more along the lines of a spiritual component of blueness that relates to a flow of water. You might notice pauses, rolling eyes, shifting in seats, facial grimaces that all suggest discomfort with any risk-taking involving listening or speaking up. Make a mental note to gently refer to such moments during the debriefing as they can be rich opportunities to flatten the hierarchy of human relationships.

> **Question:** *Why is the sky blue?*

Nurse: *The*

Nurse Manager: *sky*

Surgeon: *is*

Nurse: *blue*

Nurse Manager: *because*

Surgeon: *atmospheric*

Nurse: *fluid*

Nurse Manager: *has*

Surgeon: *provided*

Nurse: *a*

Nurse Manager: *blue*

Surgeon: *color.*

Debriefing: There are very powerful learning moments that occur in the silent moments between one person sharing a word that directs the course of the answer and the next person who is adapting to it. Invite discussion around these moments, but don't force disclosure. People are learning what they need to learn, and I encourage you to trust the process! The more you practice this approach to teaching, the more you will appreciate the power of Medical Improv.

Some questions you can use to spark discussion and reinforce experiential learning:

- What did you notice about the experience when you were part of *The Know-it-all*?
- What did you notice about the experience when you were watching or thinking of questions?

- Did anyone have to adapt to an answer going in a different way than you were thinking?
- Did anyone feel anxious about contributing a word? Can you say more about that?
- How might these experiences be helpful in your improving communication during a clinical situation?

Variation: Ideally everyone in the group will have a chance to be part of *The Know-it-all*, but you can do a demonstration with a few participants and debrief in the large group. Once participants are comfortable with the flow, you can add one or more people to the 'entity' so that there are four or five chairs with people sitting in a panel.

Notes:

Activity # 8: *This is Not a Stick* (Source unknown).

Time needed: 10 minutes

Purpose: *This is Not a Stick* is an activity that continues to build assertiveness with the added benefit of promoting creative thinking within the team. It is also a super exercise to emphasize and develop perspective-taking which is a key listening skill that has its roots in emotional intelligence. Being able to suspend judgment and honor different points of view is not easy or evident in practice much of the time. Contrary to popular opinion, being open to alternative perspectives or points of view does not require giving up or even challenging one's own opinion. Many conflicts remain unproductively stuck in power struggles because individuals are unable to see other viewpoints and are more focused on being heard rather than listening. If two or more people are defending their own points of view their ability to solve problems will be hindered.

Consider a common problem like staff that punch out for lunch, but keep on working despite management's repeated attempts to enforce meal and rest break policies. Often, in my experience, these two groups don't really understand each other's perspective and don't have the time, space, or skill to dialogue and problem-solve together. The staff nurse may worry there is not enough time in the shift to complete care, there will be negative repercussions for overtime, or they won't pick their children up from school on time. The Nurse Manager may worry about staff providing care that isn't safe or the unit not being in compliance with regulatory or budget issues. Instead of seeking solutions where all of these worries can be heard and respected, the staff nurse finds a troubling workaround.

This is Not a Stick is a great way to help professionals to internalize the notion that different perspectives are not right or wrong, they are simply different perspectives. When people don't feel so threatened by alternative thinking, they are better able to drop defenses and listen. This paves the way for more open and co-creative problem-solving.

Skills: In addition to increased communication in groups, this activity is especially helpful in promoting creativity and receptiveness to differing perspectives. As such, it is a fun way to help teams manage conflict and generate new thinking. It is also great for practicing risk-taking involved in sharing ideas and building positive energy or team spirit.

Description: Individuals in a circle pass around an object, e.g. a stick and give an example of what it could be by using it in a sentence. Participants can name anything except for what the object really is provided they come up with something different from what other participants have offered. The group should respond with any supportive comments that come to mind with each new description of the object. Change the name of the game according to the object you use, e.g. if you use an IV tube or coffee cup call the game, *This is Not an IV tube* or *This is Not a Coffee Cup* respectively.

For instance with a group of eight *This is Not a Stick* might look like this:

Person 1: *I hit a homerun with my new bat last night!*

Group responses: *Congratulations. I hear your team won the playoff. I want to borrow your bat!*

Person 2: *This corn on the cob is delicious! Would anyone to try some?* (Ok to use questions in this way!)

Group responses: *Emmmm it smells yummy. Want some butter? I'll have some!*

Person 3: *I found this dead snake outside my office!*

Group responses: *That's gross! Get it out of here. Ewwwww.*

Person 4: *There's nothing like an expensive Havana cigar!*

Group responses: *Do you have any extra? Don't light up in here. How much was it?*

Person 5: *I think this pipe will be perfect for the bathroom sink leak.*

Group responses: *Your plumbing skills are amazing. It looks perfect. YAY!*

Person 6: *I removed this giant splinter from my foot. Does anyone have a Band-Aid?*

Group responses: *That is big one. Sounds like a major operation. Wow, I hope you can walk.*

Person 7: *I'm taking my new fishing pole on vacation next week.*

Group responses: *I bet you'll catch some big ones! Can I come? Looks awesome.*

Person 8: *This IV pole extension will be good for our patients who have to have more than ten IVs going at once!*

Group responses: *You're a genious! No more tangled IV tubes. We need one on our unit.*

Facilitation: Encourage participants to add a little physical demonstration like swinging a bat or smoking a cigar. Also, look for opportunities to encourage thinking that is creative and different by giving examples. Sometimes healthcare professionals need to be reminded that it is ok to make things up and, because this is often a new way of thinking, planning on two rounds with two different objects will allow for increased comfort and risk-taking.

Debriefing: Make sure to congratulate the group on being open and able to celebrate all these different ideas. As the group finishes a round ask them which ideas were right? This is a trick question that will help bring the point home that all of the perspectives were valid. This can be used to highlight the importance of validating alternative perspectives during brainstorming and conflict management. Some additional questions you can use to spark discussion and reinforce experiential learning:

- What did you notice about the experience? Which was harder, thinking of ideas or responding to others?
- Did it get easier or harder for you to think of different ideas? What might account for any change?
- How did new and different ideas from others impact you?
- Could this object be a bat, cigar, and dead snake all at once?
- Can you still "see" the bat after someone suggests a cigar?
- How can we use this thinking when we have different opinions or ideas?
- Consider any current issues where professionals might be polarized. Is staff willing to consider alternative thinking in a more open way?

Variation: Have the group stand in a circle in an open space with the object in the middle. Take turns going into the circle and show others what the object might be such as swinging the bat. From here you can invite others to go into the circle and participate in the action going along with the bat suggestion. Someone might go in and pitch a ball or be the catcher (light the cigar, fix the sink, have some corn on the cob, etc.) With this variation, not only are different perspectives honored, but the emerging creative thought is put into action in the moment!

CHAPTER SEVEN

Notes:

Activity # 9: *Overload* (Nancy Hurley's 175 Theatre Games Warm-up Exercises for Actors).

Purpose: This is an excellent activity for team members to view stress as a part of work that impacts everyone and can lead to mistakes. One of the most positive experiences that can come from participating or observing *Overload* is a sense of comradery about the high-stakes, pressure work all team members face. This can go a long way towards reducing toxic behaviors such as judging each other about stress-related limits, (fatigue or anxiety), blaming each other for mistakes, or internalizing feelings of inadequacy about knowledge, skills, or experience. As teams shake off these old patterns of behavior they'll have more energy and ideas on how to solve problems such as unnecessary interruptions. I originally tried *Overload* with a group of healthcare professionals and theatre educators and upon observing it and subsequently teaching the activity, discovered that it can be a fun segue into practicing communication skills for improving delegation, limit-setting, giving and receiving constructive feedback, and asking for, offering, or refusing to help.

Time needed: 20 minutes

Skills: Helps with focus and concentration, increases awareness of how stress feels and looks in self and others, and promotes the understanding and honoring (in self and others) about what feels overwhelming and dangerous. This skill set is essential for working together respectfully, communicating effectively under pressure as well as building and sustaining a culture of safety.

Description: Have one person stand in the middle with the task of counting to 100 by 4s while mirroring someone standing opposite them, answering simple math questions asked by one participant on one side, and answering simple personal questions asked by the person on the other side. You can see how the activity is played with the YouTube "Interruption Awareness: A Nursing Minute for Patient Safety." [31]

Facilitation: Encourage the person mirroring to use head, arms, and torso with very slow movement that the counter can follow and is varied. In other words, movements should be simple, easy for the counter to do (in normal circumstances), very slow, and involve more than just arms and hands. You can demonstrate by turning your head,

---

[31] Beth Boynton, "Interruption Awareness: A Nursing Minute for Patient Safety." *YouTube*, uploaded January 3, 2012. https://www.YouTube.com/watch?v=PGK9_CkhRNw

bending at the waste, and waving your arms to the side and over your head. Encourage math and personal questions that under normal i.e. unstressed situations would be simple to answer.

> **Math Questioner:** *What is 3 + 2?*
>
> **Personal Questioner:** *What is your shoe size?*
>
> **Math Questioner:** *What is 7 - 3?*
>
> **Personal Questioner:** *What is your favorite kind of cereal?*

Questions should be asked at a fairly quick pace and allow for a brief pause for answers. Each round only takes 1-2 minutes so try to have as many individuals play the role of counter as possible. Be sure to honor human differences in stress responses as natural with many variables.

Debriefing: Participating in *Overload* makes the invisible yet common experience of overwhelming stress visible. As this happens it becomes more of a shared experience and that inspires compassion for self and others. This feeling of "we're in it together" is a shift that leaders and staff will appreciate and in and of itself is enough incentive to try it out! As you lead discussion notice how engaged team members become and consider how you might guide this energy towards collaborative problem-solving that regarding interruptions or other issues the team is facing. Some questions you can use to spark discussion and reinforce experiential learning:

- What did you notice about the experience as counter, mirror, etc?
- What kinds of stressors exist in the workplace?
- What individual variables influence stress levels?
- How might stress impact medical errors or sentinel events?
- What ideas do you have for minimizing stress?
- How can this activity be helpful in practicing communication skills such as setting-limits, feedback, or delegation?

Variation: Add a few other participants around the activity to provide sound effects when the counter pauses or makes a mistake. Invite ideas of common workplace sounds; such as a phone ringing, overhead page, or IV pump alarm. On occasion, some practitioners may be successful in getting to 100. This is fine, but misses the opportunity to identify one's own stress limit. You can challenge them with more interruptions or a more complex task, such as counting to 100s by 3s and skipping all even numbers or other creative ideas!

Notes:

Activity # 10: *Hitchhiker*

Time needed: 20 minutes

Purpose: *Hitchhiker* is a well-known improv activity where participants enter a pretend car with a particular attitude, mood, or behavior that the driver and passenger immediately adapt to by taking on the same attitude etc. This experience gives professionals an opportunity to feel instantly supported by the team for ideas they initiate and for team members to show collective support for the ideas. Speaking up in a group is nurtured by creating a safe environment of trusted peers who are expected to support each participant's portrayal.

Hitchhiker is a fun way to foster bonds among all members. It can be used to help shift a culture from toxic to healthy or to build cohesiveness among teams with lots of turnover or continuous changes in membership composition. In fact, it can be a fun way to show new staff how cohesive the team can be and to help welcome them.

Skills: This exercise shows how cooperation in trying new ideas and practicing a variety of attitudes, moods, and behaviors in groups; increases risk-taking and creativity in teamwork. Also, participants get instant and collective support in their risk-taking activity. This exercise can also be helpful in practicing and identifying social cues and developing empathy.

Description: Set up three chairs side by side as with *The Know-it-All*, but in this case they represent the front seat of a car. Have two volunteers take the driver's and middle seat. To start the activity, have the driver take on a particular attitude, mood, quirky behavior, or character. The passenger automatically takes on the same attitude etc. Both driver and passenger are to pretend to drive along while talking and maintaining the driver's persona until they see another participant i.e. hitchhiker and invite him or her to join them. This participant takes the third seat and starts a new conversation with a different attitude, mood, quirky behavior, or characterization. At this point, the driver and middle passenger should automatically take on the attitude etc. of the hitchhiker. The three converse in this mood while they drive along until the driver decides to stop and get out. At this point the two people in the car shift so that the middle person is now in the driver's seat and the hitchhiker's seat is now open. Now a new hitchhiker flags them down and enters the car with a new mood or persona that the others take on.

Driver (bored, yawning, speaking in low tone and sighing): *This is a pretty boring vacation.*

Middle passenger (bored, yawning, speaking in low tone and sighing): *Yeah, I'm gonna take a nap.*

Driver (bored-yawning, speaking in low tone and sighing): *I guess that is a good idea.*

Hitchhiker (anxious-flags them down gets in the car and acting anxious, e.g. speaking in quick sentences, jittery, etc. starts a conversation that is aligned with being nervous): *Oh no, I'm lost. I don't know what to do.*

Driver (now anxious): *I don't know. I took a wrong turn. Oh no!*

Middle passenger (also now anxious): *What do you mean, we're lost? I'm gonna faint. This is terrible.*

Hitchhiker (still anxious): *What is going to become of us? The world is ending!*

This can go on for a minute or two until the driver makes up a reason to stop the car, get out, and make room for a new hitchhiker with a new persona.

Facilitation: This is an activity that can start out a little stilted until people get the hang of it and feel more comfortable trying out new moods etc. Remind people of the expectation that participants respect what might or might not be comfortable for their colleagues because their choices will affect them. For the first time, I recommend you choose *Hitchhiker* characteristics that you know are safe such boring, happy, sad, rich person, poor person, person with habit of tapping their fingers; in other words, things that most people will recognize and be able to manifest, without being embarrassing or possibly pick on someone in the team. (Don't choose a quirky behavior like tapping fingers if someone in your team tends to do this unless your team is VERY cohesive and you focus on quirks that everyone has!) If you assign characteristics to each hitchhiker, this will take the pressure off for being creative or anything else that might be associated with choosing a persona. You can do this by giving each person a piece of paper with a characteristic on it or whisper to them. Or, as noted earlier, it can be fun and helpful to brainstorm a list for participants to choose from. In other words, try to keep it comfortable and safe for all participants.

I remember participating in this activity during one Medical Improv workshop and there was a male physician who was the driver and I was sitting next to him. The hitchhiker who joined us was pretending to be a woman in labor. She was screaming that her water broke and I joined right in with something along that line. This was so foreign or uncomfortable for the doctor that he couldn't do it so he kept a straight face, said nothing, and kept driving. The instructor at the time encouraged and coached him, but to no avail. In retrospect, it seemed like the degree of his discomfort was bordering on unsafe. I wondered if this could have been prevented with a little less drama and a more supportive team. On the other hand, it gave me an opportunity as a passenger to support him by pretending to see a hospital and begging him to stop and get help, which I hoped helped him to get out of the awkward situation and the activity to keep moving forward. It is a great example of how tricky maintaining a safe environment can be with applied improv.

Debriefing: Once your group is familiar with the activity, you can frame the kinds of characteristics you use to align with an organizational goal. For example, brainstorming a list of feelings common to patients and families could easily lead to great discussion and learning associated with patient experience. In this case you can you could use the activity to promote empathy and respectful communication for patients and families.

Just as profound could be a framework that lists desirable and undesirable behaviors among colleagues for creating a culture of safety. Just be careful about sensing when your group is ready for identifying and working on this kind of behavior change and if you are uncertain, it might be a good time to get some outside or leadership support! Members must be able and willing to give and receive constructive feedback. Questions you can use to spark discussion and reinforce experiential learning include:

- What did you notice about this activity?
- Which was more challenging playing the hitchhiker, driver or passenger? Say more about your experience.
- What was it like for hitchhikers when everyone took on your mood or persona?
- What, if anything, makes this activity a helpful one for building team spirit?
- How do our behaviors affect each other at work?

Variation: There are several variations of the seating, such as two seats side by side for two players, (driver and hitchhiker) or four seats side by side or creating a front and back seat with two chairs in back of two chairs. In these cases, the hitchhiker still brings the new mood or behavior to anyone else in the car.

Notes:

Now that you've helped individuals become their best selves in teams, inspired team spirit and collaborative work, and become more familiar with the experiential teaching and learning of Medical Improv, you might like to focus more on developing skills associated with leadership and followership. As mentioned earlier, there is a natural overlap of these skills for collaborative teamwork, yet as you will see there are some key differences to emphasize.

In the next chapter we'll focus on activities that help individuals become more effective leaders and followers while continuing to develop their emotional intelligence and communication skills.

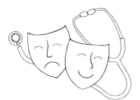

Chapter Eight: 5 Activities for Improving Leadership & Followership

There are powerful incentives to design and teach Medical Improv activities that continue to build emotional intelligence and communication skills with a leadership focus. Medical Improv can help professionals cultivate skills and build relationships, and as these examples illustrate, the leaders and followers who have demonstrated emotional intelligence and are effective and respectful communicators, will help to build healthy hierarchies and cultures of safety.

- The in-charge, authoritative surgeon who is executing commands to lead the team in highly skilled surgery and presents a demeanor that invites input from all members of the team. This is a leader who is able to articulate a vision, inspire and motivate others, guide change, manage conflict, and execute orders while being open to ideas and challenges from others.

- The confident operating room nurse who is still in training and notices that the wrong patient has been wheeled into the room and speaks up to the whole team without hesitation. This is a follower who is engaged in organizational initiatives, cooperative with change, willing to share ideas for the sake of quality improvement, and committed to carrying out and challenging orders as necessary!

Both of these professionals respect themselves and others. They are committed to using their knowledge, skills, and attitudes to provide the best patient care. Positional authority is used for clinical decision-making and there is no abuse of this power to threaten, humiliate, ignore, exclude, or withhold from others.

The activities in this chapter are designed to continue to build the emotional intelligence and communication skills that support such behaviors. In teaching them, you will help your staff explore what it feels like to lead and follow at a core level, develop empathy for the impact each has on the other, and improve competence in both areas and more. You might be surprised at how some simple activities will inspire deep reflection, dynamic discussion, and transformative individual and organizational growth!

Activity # 11: *Mirroring* (Adapted from Viola Spolin's *Theater for the Classroom*.)

Purpose: This activity will help participants gain awareness about their comfort levels as leaders and as followers with empathy for those in the other role. This kind of awareness is helpful in developing the assertiveness necessary for authoritative leadership, the ability to let someone else lead, and compassion for others who are impacted by either role. Even though some professionals, such as doctors and nurse managers will lead more than follow, developing empathy for and the capacity to follow others is essential. The same holds true for professionals who more typically will be following orders, such as nursing or physical therapy assistants, in that they should have empathy for leaders and the capacity to lead.

I remember being a preceptor for a graduate nurse who was having a hard time supervising two nursing assistants. They were requesting changes in patient assignments and permission to go on break with friends on different units. I could tell that she needed to be in charge, but wasn't comfortable with it. I motioned to her to have a private conversation. I encouraged her to be more assertive in setting limits and expressing more authority. She told me that she wasn't really seeking a leadership position and didn't believe she had the skills. I explained that being a leader was a part of what being a nurse involved and gave her some suggestions on how to handle the requests as the nurse in charge! At the time, it wasn't my role to teach Medical Improv, but looking back on it I suspect that practicing *Mirroring* would have helped this new nurse to become more confident in a leadership role and given her insights into when and why she might hesitate.

Mirroring can also help staff gain an appreciation for the idea that leading and following are not always rigid and distinct roles. The Surgical Tech who informs the Surgeon that she's about to amputate the wrong leg is a perfect example.

Time needed: 20 Minutes

Skills: Increased awareness about feelings associated with leadership and followership roles. Because many of us are more comfortable in one of these roles than the other and we must be able to do both, such awareness will help professionals develop their capacity in the areas where they need strengthening. This activity also fosters a sense of cooperation and support for leading and following and helps staff to develop empathy for those who they may lead or be led by.

Description: In pairs, participants face each other at arm's length. One person starts out as the mover (leader) and the other acts as a mirror (follower). The leader uses his or her upper body to slowly move while the other mirrors all movements. After about a minute, signal them to switch roles. This is a nonverbal activity.

Facilitation: Encourage leaders to make movements and to go at a pace that their mirror can follow successfully. After switching a couple of times ask pairs to take turns leading and following without talking and without you signaling them. Repeat the experience with another partner. Consider pairing staff with positional authority or informal power with others who are new or shy. This may be humbling to the former and empowering to the latter!

Debriefing: Encourage everyone to try to step out of their comfort zone and reassure participants that it is normal for people to feel more comfortable with one role or the other. It can be very challenging for some on either side of the continuum, who may feel very uncomfortable with sharing power, and it is important to be sensitive to this. You can always allow for some to simply observe, if they appear resistant. In such situations, they will still be learning some powerful insights about their own behavior. Some questions you can use to spark discussion and reinforce experiential learning:

- What did you notice about the experience?
- Did anyone feel more comfortable in one role versus the other? Share more! What might make it easier or harder?
- Did your comfort level with leading or following influence the activity when switching roles was self-determined? If so, how?
- What differences, if any, did you notice when switching partners?
- Did anyone lose track of who was leading at any points?

- How do leaders support followers in this activity?
- How do followers support leaders?
- How can this experience help you in your work or with your career?

Variation: After pairs get comfortable with *Mirroring,* have two pairs become a quad and chose leaders by tapping one on the shoulder. Have quads form a group of eight and tap different people one by one to lead. Alternatively and without music, form circles of 10 or so. Ask everyone to identify someone to mirror by pointing or nodding. This time tell participants not to initiate anything purposefully and just allow for mirroring to take place naturally. I've experienced this with groups and there seems to be a team energy that evolves and sometimes everyone is doing the same motion. It is hard to tell who is leading or following and can be a very pleasant closure activity. Also, if you want to focus on making the hierarchy more flexible, this circle mirroring variation can spur some great discussion about shared responsibility in leading and following! If you are curious to learn more and apply this activity differently, you might enjoy searching the internet with "follow the follower in improv". This is a term used in improvisation that refers to leadership and followership as a process with less distinct roles.

Notes:

Activity # 12: *Cars* (Source unknown).

Purpose: This activity is designed to build trust between participants and provide opportunities to discover what it is like to control others or be controlled by others. As much as I am a proponent of collaborative leadership and flattening the hierarchy, there are very important reasons for maintaining a ladder of authority. Education, knowledge, and clinical experience are all good reasons for doctors to give orders to nurses that nurses should follow. The same is true for Physical Therapists giving orders to Physical Therapy Assistants, Nurses to Nurse Assistants, and Occupational Therapists to Occupational Therapy Assistants. Knowing when and how to exert authority is an essential skill and learning how it impacts others can help leaders to be more compassionate and respectful when doing so.

This activity helps professionals experience how their feelings about power influence their leadership decisions. Such awareness is essential to filter out self-serving motives from those geared towards safe and cost-effective care. The same can be said for followers, who might not pursue leadership paths because their own, albeit different feelings about power keep them from taking on authoritative roles that they are well prepared for otherwise.

Time needed: 20 minutes

Skills: Builds trust, creates focus on the relationship between leaders and followers and the vulnerability and responsibilities that are included in them; and provides opportunity to practice both roles. The activity can be used to develop empathy for patients or others feeling a loss of control. Also, increasing the number of pairs working in the same place can be helpful in developing situational awareness and challenges associated with it.

Description: Work in open space in pairs with one person being the driver and the other person being the car. The driver faces the back of the person being the car using their dominant hand to instruct the car:

- Palm on upper back signals "go straight forward".
- Palm removed signals "stop".
- Fingers to top of right shoulder signals "turn to right".
- Fingers to top of left shoulder signals "turn to left".

This is a nonverbal activity.

Facilitation: Make sure there is enough space for pairs to move about the room. You can start with two or three pairs moving about and then add more pairs depending on space. Instruct pairs to speed up and slow down a couple of times. Make sure to switch roles. Encourage participants to try being both the driver and the car even if it feels that one or the other roles are very unlikely in their day to day work. It may help to reinforce the empathy-building component of the experience before, during, and after the activity. Observing this activity can be helpful and remember that a participant who resists an activity will already be gaining insight about their own behavior. Maintaining a safe environment is the priority!

Debriefing: In order to be sensitive about insecurities that might arise with discussion and reflection, it may help to imagine a surgeon having a hard time playing the role of a car especially if the car is driven by a nurse who is new to the operating room team. It may feel like a threat to the surgeon's ego. It might be equally challenging for the new nurse. Keep in mind that the philosophy behind teaching Medical Improv is to help all professionals grow and to create a safe environment for doing so. This makes it important to nudge participants to discuss and reflect but not force.

Some questions you can use to spark discussion and reinforce experiential learning:

- What did you notice about the experience?
- Which role did you like or feel more comfortable in, car or driver?
- Can you think of times at work when you must be one role and at other times, the other? What helps you to be more successful?
- How important is trust in this activity? Say more!
- Where does the power to control come from? In this activity? In clinical situations?
- What responsibilities do leaders have in using power?
- How can you use this experience to become a more effective leader, follower, or more compassionate professional?

Variation: Have participants close their eyes. This will increase dependency and can relate back to building trust and empathy. You can also add commands:

- Increased pressure of palm to back signals "increase speed".
- Decreased pressure of palm to back signals "decrease speed".
- Finger poke to mid back signals car to "Honk"!

As adding these commands gives the drivers more control, this can be a focus in your debriefing. Another way to use this activity is to have more pairs in the space at the same time, which will pave the way for discussion and learning that will promote situational awareness.

Notes:

Activity # 13: *Status Walk* (Adapted from Viola Spolin's *Theater for the Classroom*.)

Purpose: *Status Walk* will help participants become familiar with what verbal and nonverbal behaviors of high and low status look, feel, and sound like. In preparing you'll want to be familiar with them:

People with High Status

- Speak clearly and audibly
- Use few words
- Seem comfortable with silence
- Never apologize
- Stand with legs apart and strong, open shoulders/arms taking up a lot of space
- Sit back in chair relaxed, confident, and in charge
- Seek out eye contact
- Maintain confidence even when not making sense

People with Low Status

- Speak softly and mutter
- Use a lot of words
- Feel uncomfortable with silence
- Apologize a lot
- Hunch shoulders and take up less physical space
- Use a lot of anxious gestures like covering mouth and fidgeting
- Squirm in chair or sit on the edge, generally uncomfortable sitting
- Avoid eye contact
- Retract statements even when making sense
- Use facial expressions that indicate doubt, anxiety and/or low self-esteem

Professionals will be able to use status in helpful and therapeutic ways and correct behavior that is more destructive. These examples show how status behavior can be helpful:

- A doctor uses an authoritative and directive tone in dictating the code team's response to a patient's cardiac arrest.
- A nurse uses assertive tone and body language while raising concerns with a

physician about a patient's clinical status.
- A nurse's assistant sits down next to a patient with dementia while feeding him.
- A nurse practitioner speaks softly and is mindful of his body posture in order to lower his status and create psychological safety for an anxious patient.

Unfortunately, we can also all likely attest to seeing status used inappropriately or worse, in ways that interfere with safe care and optimal patient experience. For example:

- A nurse apologizes frequently, mutters, and covers her mouth when raising concerns about a patient's clinical status.
- A doctor uses dismissive and humiliating language to belittle a nurse who raised concerns about a patient's clinical status.
- A physician assistant assumes that her knowledge of the side effects of a medication is superior to a patient's and discounts the patient's report.
- A nurse's assistant doesn't knock before entering a patient's room.

This can be a very illuminating activity to do because high and low status behaviors are going on all the time without us realizing it. With awareness, staff will have all sorts of opportunities to use status behaviors in positive ways!

Time needed: 30 Minutes

Skills: Increased awareness of verbal and nonverbal behaviors associated with high and low status and the feelings associated with both; creates opportunities to discuss helpful and unhelpful (or hurtful) use of status behaviors in leadership and followership with colleagues and patients.

Description: Have the group walk around the space as if they are in a business meeting and all have high status. They can talk with each other. Then have them do the same thing as if they all have low status. After this, have half the group be high and the other half low and walk around in the meeting together.

Facilitation: Encourage participants to use their posture, facial expressions, and verbal tone to show that they are very high or very low status. Invite them to genuinely feel what each status is like. Allow for a minute or so for each walk around.

Debriefing: It is important to facilitate discussion that includes the expressions of high and low status mentioned earlier. You can do that as a lead-in into the activity or with the debriefing. The advantage of doing it beforehand is that it will bring out more ideas about behaviors. Since status behaviors are going on all the time, consciously and unconsciously, most expressions will occur spontaneously when participants are asked to demonstrate them.

Some questions you can use to spark discussion and reinforce experiential learning:

- How did it feel to be in the high status group vs. the low status group? Was one more comfortable than the other?
- Can you express a high or low status even if you don't feel comfortable doing so?
- How is status related to leadership or followership?
- How is status used in helpful vs. unhelpful ways with colleagues and patients?
- What ways can you envision using these status behaviors in helpful ways in clinical situations?

You can also use the examples with status that I've listed for role-plays or for challenging the group to identify helpful vs. unhelpful status behaviors.

Variation: If you have a big enough group you can have 8-10 participants walk around in high status while the others are tasked with observing for verbal and nonverbal behaviors that signify it. After a minute or so ask the audience to share their observations and then do the same for low status. You can also plan to revisit the debriefing after some time. This will help reinforce learning that happened during the activity and also make room for sharing additional insights that occur as participants make new observations at work.

Status activities can lead to lots of discussion and reflection that continues to raise awareness over time. There are lots of ways you can build on status activities that lead to fascinating explorations into human behaviors. Doing these activities and then searching the internet and/or looking through additional resources for more along with the discussions sparked in your sessions will likely give you some new ideas. Potential topics include: developing empathy for people who hold different levels of status, exploring how social or cultural mores define status, or discussing how status and power influence human behavior! And because healthcare inherently involves human beings and relationships, the relevance to our work seems unlimited. As you become more experienced with and knowledgeable about teaching Medical Improv and gain insights into staff behavior, interests, and needs, you'll find all sorts of possible applications!

Notes:

Activity # 14: *Columbian Hypnosis*-Adapted from Augusta Baol's Games for Actors and Non-actors[32]

Purpose: *Columbian Hypnosis*, like *Mirroring*, will help participants gain awareness about their comfort levels as leaders and as followers and empathy for others in the other role. It is another activity for developing assertiveness necessary for authoritative leadership; the ability to let someone else lead; and compassion for others who are impacted by the other role. It can help leaders at all levels to become more flexible and competent with all leadership styles. Unlike *Mirroring*, the leadership is more authoritative and unlike *Cars* the followership is more adaptive, i.e human. These differences allow for some interesting reflections and discussions about having, using, and sharing power.

Since many organizations are shifting towards cultures of safety that are more collaborative, this activity can be used to engage staff in the work of culture change. Without looking at the many variations, you can simply use the activity to demonstrate the old ways of authoritative-only leadership. In fact, there are so many potential variations, I encourage you to teach the activity a few times in order to see how it unfolds and try it out yourself. In doing so, I suspect you will appreciate the variations even more and come up with a few of your own that will help your team and organizational goals in unique ways.

Time needed: 20 Minutes

Skills: Raising awareness about what it feels like to act as an authoritative leader and to be a follower of this leadership style. You can focus on either or both with varying group sizes. In addition to strengthening abilities in and empathy for both roles, the fluid nature of collaborative leadership and teamwork can be explored at a deep level. Also, with variations in the activity, situational awareness, change management the complexity of leadership, relationships, and trust can be explored and developed.

Description: In pairs, the palm of one person's hand (Person A) hand is held 6-8 inches

---

[32] Augusto Boal, *Games for Actors and Non-Actors*, trans. Adrian Jackson, New York, Routledge, 2002

away from person B's face as if hypnotizing their partner to follow the palm wherever it goes. Person B should maintain the 6-8 inch distance while person A leads person B to bend and turn and walk slowly around the room. After a couple of minutes the roles are switched. After both partners have played each role, instruct the pairs to lead and follow (hypnotize each other) at the same time. This is a nonverbal activity.

Facilitation: Encourage leaders to be mindful of the physical limitations of others as they push their palm forward and back, side to side, up and down as well as leading partners around the room. Alternatively, you can frame the activity with instruction that includes, "Be gentle and reasonable with physical gestures because we all have limits", or begin by having partners exchange any physical limitations by having them hold a brief conversation. I suggest giving an example, such as stating, "I have an old knee injury". Encourage followers to keep their eyes focused on their leaders palm and maintain the distance as best they can.

Debriefing: Some questions you can use to spark discussion and reinforce experiential learning:

- What did you notice about the activity?
- How did it feel to be the leader versus follower? Was one more comfortable or easier?
- What was it like when you were doing both?
- How can this experience help you grow as an individual?
- How does this kind of leadership manifest in healthcare? Are there any positive or negative repercussions?
- Did this experience give you any insights about your role as a leader or follower?
- How can this experience help you become a more effective leader or follower?

Variation: There are all sorts of variations to this activity and if you search the internet for videos on it, you'll find lots of examples. Try having one leader, using both palms, with a different follower for each palm. Have one (or both) of those followers use one of their palms to hypnotize a fourth person (and/or fifth). Be creative about adding more followers and having those followers be leaders for one or two others while having others make observations about behaviors and skills.

If you are familiar with complexity science, the variations of this activity offer a fun way to explore leadership and followership within complex adaptive systems such as healthcare professionals in teams and organizations! You can also have one leader with a group of followers. Have followers stand a foot or two from the leader's palm.You can create a model of a complex adaptive system by explaining the leader's palm is the vision of the organization and the group of six or more followers must follow a few rules, much like a flock of birds heading south! Instruct the followers to keep their eyes on the leader's palm and:

1. Avoid collisions with others.
2. Match speeds with neighbors
3. Move toward the center of the group.

At any moment you can direct another person from the group or audience to take on the leadership role while having the rest of the group including the former leader adapt to the new leader. Once you and your group become familiar with this activity, you can be creative over time with it's application. For example, you can assign an intention to the leader such as controlling versus visionary, or assign an intention to a group to be cooperative or resistant. These types of activities can open the door to discussions around informal power, leadership styles, and organizational vision.

Notes:

Activity # 15: *Gibberish Talk Show* (Adapted from Kat Koppett's *Training to Imagine*)

Purpose: In *Gibberish Talk Show* there is an interdependence of three people who impact each other's roles in the creation of 'scene'. This is a great activity for demonstrating how everyone plays an important role in outcomes or if you are trying to break down 'silos' between departments or shifts. It is a fun way to help people understand that they need each other in order to provide the best care and to explore working together more collaboratively.

For example, if bickering between shifts on a nursing unit is affecting morale, patient care, and use of resources, (which it probably is) consider using this activity as part of ongoing unit meetings. If it is feasible to have some nurses from each shift at the meeting, you can encourage their participation and they will experience sharing leadership and followership responsibilities and appreciating each other's role. This can ripple out into everyday dynamics and over time and subsequent meetings involve more nurses.

Teaching and playing *Gibberish Talk Show* is a little more challenging than other activities, but once some of your staff get the knack of gibberish and the flow of the activity, it will become easier for you and them!

Time needed: 20 minutes

Skills: This activity provides an opportunity to develop creativity in both leading and following roles. It is lots of fun to watch. The time needed above will allow for you to introduce the activity, do it once, and debrief. Because this activity involves three participants with all others watching, it has the added risk and benefit of developing public speaking skills.

Description: Three volunteers sit in front of the group decide who is going to play the role of Talk Show Host, Expert, and Translator. The Talk Show Host speaks and understands only English (or the primary language of the group). The Expert, understands English, but only speaks her own language, i.e. gibberish (a made up language unique to each improviser). The Translator speaks and understands both languages. This allows the Expert to answer questions directly from the Talk Show Host and the Translator to translate the Expert's answers (and not the questions). Once this concept is understood, you or the participants come up with a topic that the Expert pretends to be the world's leading authority on. The Talk Show Host will ask the Expert questions in English, the Expert will answer in Gibberish, and the Translator will explain what the Expert says!

It can be a little confusing at first but well worth the effort as once people get the concept of Gibberish and understand their roles; the interdependence is a rich source of learning. In the following example, the topic is "wine tasting" and you can introduce the show something like this:

> **Facilitator:** *Welcome to Marvin Salter Show live from Hollywood. Today's guest, the world famous wine taster, Falecia Cabernet. Joining Falecia to translate for us is Joseph Russell.*
>
> **Talk Show Host:** *Hi folks and welcome Falecia.*
>
> **Expert:** *Cloosara mefinto.*
>
> **Translator:** *I'm delighted to be here.*
>
> **Talk Show Host:** *Can you tell us a little bit about how you got started in wine-tasting?*
>
> **Expert:** *Ahhhh, sompito. Clunedepin stosaploffy conefeson fundeplep. Tonsoro flendusen clopsinger.*
>
> **Translator:** *Of course. When I was a little girl, my father used to grow grapes and sell them in the market. I used to love to help him pick the grapes. Everything was fine until the fire.*
>
> **Talk Show Host:** *The fire? Can you tell us about that?*

Facilitation: It can be helpful to have the Expert use an accent to help with their gibberish or the audience can provide one. If German was selected the above conversation might sound more like this:

> **Talk Show Host:** *Hi folks and welcome Falecia.*
>
> **Expert:** *Mein flinkenstien schweppen!*

Translator: *I'm delighted to be here.*

Talk Show Host: *Can you tell us a little bit about how you got started in wine-tasting?*

Expert: *Ahhhh, Das Klengenmitz fundhoffer. Und spletzenfein gesundenfaltz zind leebshenduggen.*

Translator: *Of course. When I was a little girl, my father used to grow grapes and sell them in the market. I used to love to help him pick the grapes. Everything was fine until the fire.*

Talk Show Host: *The fire? Can you tell us about that?*

Encourage the Expert to use nonverbal cues to help guide the story. Encourage the Translator to use the tone and body language from the Expert to help guide the story and to add their own ideas. Also, let the Talk Show Host know that he can create questions that also steer the story. For example:

Talk Show Host: *I read in your book that the fire was devastating to your family and that you have nightmares to this day? Can you tell us about that?*

After a few questions, invite the Talk Show Host to ask the rest of the group if they have any questions. Part of the magic of this activity is that each of the three people share in the creation of the story. The observers can help direct the story too by asking questions. In terms of leadership and followership in collaborative work, everyone has power!

Debriefing: Some questions you can use to spark discussion and reinforce experiential learning:

- What did each of the players notice about their role and the story?
- What did the observers notice?
- What does this activity teach us about collaboration between shifts or departments?
- What does this activity teach us about verbal and nonverbal communication

and its role in teamwork and leadership?
- Could use of jargon be perceived as Gibberish by patients? How might this impact their feelings of power or our efforts to provide patient-centered care?

Variation: Try having a job interview, where the interviewee for a position as a Sous Chef speaks Gibberish or a news reporter interviewing an astronaut about her trip to Mars. Feel free to alter the details of job position or news event! Another way to use Gibberish is to have one person teach how to do something or sell a product to the rest of the group while one other person translates into English.

Notes:

Conclusion

I hope that you and your staff are enjoying your experiences with Medical Improv, in developing essential skills, having a positive impact on patient safety, patient experience, and workforce health, while having fun together!

As a student or teacher, it can be awkward or even scary to try something so different! Congratulations to you and your staff for stepping out of your comfort zone to do work that is so critical to the care you provide, the patients you serve, and the satisfaction you feel for playing an important part in the healthcare system.

I hope that this Primer and these activities have provided you with a new, effective, and fun alternative to building essential skills. As the field of Medical Improv continues to emerge, please share your successes, challenges, and new ideas with your colleagues and me!

Beth

Beth@bethboynton.com

CHAPTER EIGHT | 149

Afterword

By Stephanie Frederick, RN, M.Ed.

Beth Boynton walks her talk.

We met at the first Medical Improv training, developed and taught by Katie Watson at Chicago's Northwestern University. Beth and I have extensive RN experience, and immediately recognized the potential for using Medical Improv in clinical and educational settings. She has ensured that the value of Medical Improv is understood in this primer, and the basics are accessible and affordable to a wide range of healthcare professionals and organizations.

Quality of care, patient safety, and workforce health are three issues Beth has chosen to focus on. Her years in organizational development qualify her to speak, practice, and write about how communication, relationships, and behaviors are linked to health care issues. Medical Improv and Beth are an empowered, dynamic duo!

I feel exhilarated by the FUN and laughter that accompany the Medical Improv workshops I've facilitated. It's not standup comedy; it's about connection and communication. When's the last time you had FUN and felt tuned in to your creativity at a healthcare conference? My guess is that it hasn't happened, and that's why this primer, with the accompanying descriptive exercises, is written for all of us.

I encourage you to focus on the power of Improvisational Theater's core principles. *Yes, and...*, *help your partner be successful*, *you have everything you need*, *celebrate risk-taking*, *truth and facts are not necessary*, *avoid questions,* and *observers play an important role*. Everyone is energized when the focus is on listening, sharing ideas, and supporting others. It's inspiring to hear workshop feedback about the awe of engaging with other participants, regardless of rank, status, education, or department. All are invited, and everyone is encouraged to participate!

Medical Improv workshops generate a lot of enthusiasm, and most people are anxious to get back to their work environments and share the lessons. Until now that's been a difficult thing to do. Beth's primer is a priceless addition to learn and practice the skills with a colleague, a group of folks, or your entire organization. She will answer any additional questions you have, and is always willing to collaborate. She's the supreme connector!

Medical Improv is shifting the culture of healthcare with the emotional intelligence that ensures quality patient care and holistic health for employees. By practicing the skills Beth has introduced in this primer, you and your colleagues will experience enriched communication and collaboration. The patients we care for will ultimately benefit. We all know it's time to do things differently. I invite you to go out and spread the word!

Stephanie Frederick, RN, MEd
Improv to Improve Healthcare!
www.stephaniefrederick.com